GRAHAM PASSEY

LOOKING
FOR THE
Rainbow

The Sally Painting Story

GRAHAM PASSEY

LOOKING
FOR THE
Rainbow

The Sally Painting Story

MEREO
Cirencester

Mereo Books

1A The Wool Market Dyer Street Cirencester Gloucestershire GL7 2PR
An imprint of Memoirs Publishing www.mereobooks.com

Looking for the Rainbow: 978-1-86151-418-9

First published in Great Britain in 2015
by Mereo Books, an imprint of Memoirs Publishing

The address for Memoirs Publishing Group Limited can be found at
www.memoirspublishing.com

The Memoirs Publishing Group Ltd Reg. No. 7834348

The Memoirs Publishing Group supports both The Forest Stewardship Council® (FSC®) and
the PEFC® leading international forest-certification organisations. Our books carrying both the
FSC label and the PEFC® and are printed on FSC®-certified paper. FSC® is the only
forest-certification scheme supported by the leading environmental organisations including
Greenpeace. Our paper procurement policy can be found at
www.memoirspublishing.com/environment

Typeset in 13/18pt Bembo
by Wiltshire Associates Publisher Services Ltd. Printed and bound in Great Britain by
Printondemand-Worldwide, Peterborough PE2 6XD

CONTENTS

Foreword

Introduction

FOREWORD

❧

This book has been in Graham Passey's mind for the last eight years, born out of every husband's and parent's nightmare. On the Feast of the Conversion of St Paul (25 January) 2005, Sally Painting's firstborn, Edward, died shortly after his premature birth. Some twelve hours later, Sally too died, leaving her distraught husband, Mike, her parents Val and Graham and brothers Andrew and Robert.

From an early age, Sally had kept a daily diary. It is a straightforward, everyday account of activities in Sally's life. By the time she started her diary it was known Sally had a diseased liver and biopsies and gastroscopies were to become a regular part of her routine, recorded in her diary as everyday events alongside comments about school and home life. What is startling about her record is the ordinariness with which this remarkable young lady wrote about her quite extraordinary life.

During her teenage years, Sally struggled with her studies as she endured continuing treatment for her chronic illness, including the emergency removal of her spleen and later, a significant part of her intestines. Yet she persevered, qualifying as a nurse and, uniquely, becoming a sister on the very unit where, at the age of 19, she had received a transplanted liver. Perhaps we can imagine the impact Sally had on patients who, terrified at the prospect of such a major event as a liver transplant, found the nurse in charge of their care to be someone who had herself undertaken such a journey.

In this book, Graham has collated Sally's diaries to tell her story from the one authentic viewpoint – Sally's. Reflecting on the discovery of diaries from a nineteenth-century inhabitant of The Cottage, Sally's home until her marriage to Mike, Sally muses whether someone in the future will be interested in her diaries. The answer to that must be "Thank you, Sally, for writing them, for giving us further insight into the young lady who quietly, almost ordinarily, exhibited such enormous and extraordinary personal strength and faith."

Many readers of this book will have had the

privilege of knowing Sally, Mike and the rest of her family. You will know just what a loving and self-giving family they are. This book – and the risk of writing it - exudes Graham's love for his only daughter. It is an act of love. Thank you, Graham, for this gift of love, for sharing with us your personal journey into the depths of despair brought on by your love for Sally. This is the mystery of what it is to be truly human, a mystery worked out on the Cross of Calvary 2,000 years ago when Jesus, fully man, in the depths of a despair brought on by God's love for the world, revealed, in his divinity, the divine potential in us all.

The Revd Canon Peter Holliday | Lichfield, November 2014

INTRODUCTION

Sally had an affinity for rainbows, the classic biblical symbol of hope; that the sunshine will always follow the rain. Or, as Genesis 9. v16 says 'Whenever the rainbow appears in the clouds, I will see it and remember the everlasting covenant between God and all living creatures of every kind on earth.'

Sally kept a daily diary from the age of ten and these have provided wonderful insights into her innermost thoughts and been a rich source of material in writing this book.

And my claim to fame? I am Sally's dad.
This is Sally's story.

Graham Passey | January 2015

CHAPTER ONE

I'VE SEEN HER, AND SHE IS BEAUTIFUL

❧

1974-79

Monday 7ᵗʰ October 1974
'Dad is sleeping soundly. Mum is starting to wonder if these funny feelings are the start of contractions. This is the day I will be born. How unprepared they seem to be. They even think that their first-born will be a son, so I don't even have a name yet! How little do they realise how I will change their lives forever.'

Val rouses me from my slumbers; she seems to think that this is it and we should get a move on. We get up quietly. The hospital bag is all prepared – spare clothes, camera, pack of cards etc .We wake my mum, who is staying with us while her own home is refurbished, and she also thinks we should get a move on. It's bound to be ages yet.

We get to the hospital and Val is settled into a little room while I am despatched to a very smoky waiting room. Eventually I am allowed back and we start our game of cards, which is interrupted from time to time to check on Val's progress. I wait outside or in the smoky room. We are almost certain it will be a boy, to be called Andrew, but just in case, we ought to have a girl's name ready. There is a song in the top twenty called 'Sally Sunshine.' I had always liked the name Sally (I was a fan of Gracie Fields as a boy but I didn't say much about it at school!)

Jane was the second name of my maternal grandmother so, in the unlikely event of it being a girl, Sally Jane Passey it will be.

The interruptions get more regular (to do with more regular contractions). I am asked to go to the waiting room once more. I really must make it clear whether or not I wish to attend the birth (I really should). It has been a long time. Has the nurse forgotten to tell me I can go back?

I creep back to find the room empty. Where on earth can she be? A further long wait before Sister Mavis Orton (someone we knew very well, as she was a member of our local church) walks down the corridor to the smoky room and says 'Have they told you?'

'Have they told me what?'

'You have a lovely baby daughter.'

'Are you sure?' is all I can think to say.

'Oh yes' she says, 'I've seen her, and she is beautiful'.

And she was!

So, Sally Jane it was.

I returned home in the car that night singing 'Sally Sunshine' at the top of my voice. The mixture of relief that all was well, and sheer elation at becoming a father, made it the happiest day of my life.

Val and Sally came out of hospital ten days later (very different from the norm these days) and we were able to properly show her off to family and friends.

Sally was such a happy baby, always smiling and laughing. Both grandmothers were able to enjoy their first grandchild, and Val's dad was over the moon and proud as punch. The birth gave my mum a much-needed boost as my dad had passed away in March of the previous year, after a long struggle with lung cancer.

Within twelve months Sally had been to two weddings. The first, in April 1975, was that of Val's brother, Peter, and his bride, Joan. I was able to reciprocate as best man to Peter, as he had been my best man in August 1970.

In September my brother, Eric, was married to Sue on a beautiful sunny day. I vividly remember my mum proudly holding a very smiley Sally.

Mum had been diagnosed with stomach cancer in the spring and had an operation followed by chemo and radiotherapy. She had made a supreme effort to be at Eric's wedding, sporting a wig. It was a great comfort for her to learn that Val was pregnant again but sadly, she would not survive to see her second grandchild. It became necessary for Mum to move in with us again, this time to be cared for. She died on December 5th, aged 58, when Sally was 14 months old.

1976/77

Val had hoped to have our second child at home but when he (surely it would be a boy this time?) threatened to arrive very early, she was required to be confined to bed in hospital for three weeks. I thoroughly enjoyed looking after Sally at home during this time, with the help of Val's mum and dad. After a week I was allowed to take Sally into hospital to see Val, but only in the day room. Sally transfixed Val in her new red dress and shoes, which I had enjoyed buying for her.

Andrew Francis was eventually born on time on the 21st April 1976, the Queen's 50th birthday. Sally enjoyed helping to look after her little brother and was soon pushing him round in the 'toddle truck'. Andrew was very content with this and saw no reason to start to walk very much until he was 16 months old.

1978/79

We soon began thinking of moving to a larger family house and after several abortive attempts, found a beautiful 500-year-old cottage in the village of Longdon, about fifteen miles away. We first saw the house on a lovely sunny day in May 1979. We were so taken with it that we returned the next day and agreed to buy it.

The owners were looking to buy their next house at auction, so we agreed to complete when they found one. In the event it took six months, so Sally had to start school at Florendine Street in Amington for a few weeks. We eventually completed the purchase and moved in November of that year.

I fondly remember Sally and Andrew running round the kitchen table late at night on the day we moved in, excited at the extra space to run around in. I think we were all too excited to sleep.

We soon settled to village life and Sally immediately started at the primary school in the village. The day after we moved in we went to the church garden fete at Longdon School. Sally started her new school the following week, Andrew started the playgroup and Val joined the WI! In due course Sally joined the local Brownies and made new friends.

CHAPTER TWO

JOY - AND DEVASTATION

∝∝∝

1980-82

In January 1980, we bought a Border Collie puppy and named her Sadie. The children were thrilled with their first real pet and enjoyed taking her for walks in the local countryside. This new member of the family, however, proved not to be enough, and the following year Val was pregnant again.

At the start of the autumn term, Sally was feeling generally unwell. She felt tired, lethargic and unhappy and was away from school. Our local midwife, Winnie, was visiting Val and noticed that Sally appeared to be jaundiced. We hadn't noticed - we had just thought she had a sun tan from our recent summer holiday.

After a visit to our doctor and a referral to a liver specialist, Sally underwent a series of blood tests and a liver biopsy, resulting in a diagnosis of non-A, non-B chronic active hepatitis. We did not initially fully understand the serious implications of this, but the news triggered many visits to different hospitals for tests and treatment.

After threatening to arrive early, Robert Graham arrived on time on 18th January, a healthy 8 lb 10 oz. Sally, at almost eight years old, was quite capable of helping with baby and soon became his second mum.

In 1982, as Sally approached her eighth birthday, Val kept a holiday diary for a few weeks. It was the year when Sally began a series of many different hospital visits for endless blood tests, scans, x-rays and liver biopsies. Sally always approached these with great courage and fortitude, but we found them very troubling, concerned about where the tests were leading.

Thursday 5th August
Overcast start to a sultry day. Delightfully spent over at Tamworth open-air pool with the children and Anne Garratt and her children, Rachel and Andrew. The pool was quiet and we enjoyed a warm swim and a picnic prepared by Anne. Sally and Andrew are very confident in the water now. They jumped in and went down the slide many times. I think this was the best day of the holiday for them. It is strange to think that I was Sally's age when I first went to Tamworth pool. Winnie, the midwife, popped in after visiting Judy and her new baby, next door. A terrible storm after tea. Andrew has a craze on butterflies and keeps a caterpillar in a jar.

Friday 6th August
Great excitement that the caterpillar has eaten much of a nettle leaf and is getting fat. Robert has developed a quaint way of rocking backwards and forwards. Andrew and Sally went to Kathryn Ellis's first birthday party. Sally made the cake. They both enjoyed the party and came home with felt pens. Sally is enjoying writing her holiday diary. Bad news that Sally's blood tests were not too good.

Monday 9th August
Graham starts a one-week holiday. Started the day at Bucknall Hospital with Sally having her 8th blood test. She was very brave. I don't know how I feel, as she has to go in for a liver biopsy. The rest of the day was spent at Alton Towers, where Sally and Andrew certainly got their money's worth.

Tuesday 10th August
As Sally is going to Bucknall Hospital at bedtime, we thought it best to have a jolly good day. This we did by taking a picnic to Tamworth outdoor pool. Granddad met us there and we all had a good swim. Robert watched and Andrew played crazy golf.

Wednesday 11th August
Sally had a liver biopsy. We went to see her in the afternoon I was very troubled.

Thursday 12th August
It was lovely to have Sally home in the afternoon. The biopsy has taken away her strength, but I think a good night's sleep should see some improvement.

Wednesday 18th August
Robert is 7 months old today. It was lovely to hear him say 'Daddy'. Andrew is still interested in caterpillars and is playing with Carl in the lane. Sally is looking after Sue Ryder's cat - competently opening the food tins and locking the doors etc.

Friday 20th August
A very gruelling day. We took Sally to Stoke Royal Infirmary for an isotope scan. We then went to Bucknall Hospital, where she had a sweat test and urine sample. Dr Tubbs had a long chat with us. He explained certain tests that ought to be carried out. We both feel devastated.

Tuesday 24th August
We took Sally to Stoke City General Hospital for a barium meal and many x-rays.

Friday 3rd September
We both took Sally to Bucknall Hospital for a glucose test.

Friday 8th October
We both took Sally to London. Spent the morning sight-seeing before our appointment at Kings College Hospital to see Dr Mowatt, a liver specialist.

After the visit we were asked to take part in a nationwide study of families where one member had liver disease. Sally's 8th birthday was on the 7th October and we celebrated with a party on the Saturday. A welcome relief after a difficult week.

Sally's last two years at primary school, 1983/84

The year started with further hospital visits and tests, including a one-night stay at Bucknall Hospital. Sally always bore these stoically but we were getting increasingly concerned. She was also put on a course of steroids which had the effect of making her beautiful face a lot fatter.

Sally always enjoyed taking a full part in village activities including brownies, assisting with the crèche at church, and baking cakes for the annual produce show. She also inherited her mum's abilities with all sorts of craft activities, including sewing and embroidery.

On her 10th birthday we hosted a 'posh' dinner for a group of her girl friends, and I donned my dinner suit to serve as head waiter.

Starting a diary, 1985

This is the first entry in Sally's first diary, in which every day she would faithfully record the triumphs and the tragedies, the miraculous and the mundane:

Tuesday 1st January
Today we all went for a walk and a picnic to Milford Hills. Grandma and Granddad came as well. We had a nice time. Later I watched a James Bond film (Dr No) and also Knight Riders (Stunts). That was ACE.

Tuesday 8th January
Today at school we had Robert Ellis to take our assembly. When I got home I wrote a letter to Jimmy Savile to see if he could fix it for me to go to the laboratory to see my blood being tested.

Thankfully Sally never received a reply to this request.

Wednesday 9th January
Today at 7.00am Mum woke me up and at 7.30am Dad

took me to Pokey Stokey (Bucknall Hospital, Stoke on Trent). When I got there this doctor felt my tummy and he hurt me. Then he said 'WHAT DID YOU HAVE FOR CHRISTMAS?' and I said 'my skirt' and then Dad said 'and your watch.' Then the doctor said 'CAN YOU TELL THE TIME THEN?' and I said 'yes', thinking 'WHAT A BANANA!'

This is the first entry in the diary referring to the many early morning trips to Bucknall Hospital for blood tests and examinations, since Doctor Tubbs had diagnosed a particular rare form of hepatitis known as 'non-A non-B chronic non-contagious hepatitis'. Sally stoically put up with all the various tests and examinations, including very painful procedures to obtain a specimen of the liver on which to perform a biopsy.

Within three years we were to have devastating news about the seriousness of her condition.

Friday 18th January -
Robert's 3rd birthday
Today, when I woke up, I took Robert's present into mum's room (Dad's room as well!) and he opened it. It was a Mr Man book (Mr Wrong). Mum and Dad bought him a wheelbarrow. At teatime Robert had a party. Sarah Grew, Sarah White, Kathryn Ellis and Alex Passey came. They all had a great time.

Saturday 2nd February

Dad's 40th birthday

Today it was Dad's birthday and when he came down the stairs there was his BIG present under a sheet. It was a BIKE and Dad liked it. At about half past eleven in the morning Dad and I went for a 5-mile bike ride. When we got back home we all went to the pub for lunch. After lunch I went swimming with Marie. Then I went back to Marie's house to stay the night. We had a really brill time.

Wednesday 27th February

Today Mum took me to Stoke-on–Trent (Bucknall Hospital) to have a check-up. Dr Tubbs felt my tummy and then gave me a blood test. When I had finished at the hospital, Mum and I went to Uttoxeter and did a little bit of shopping. We bought curtain material for Andrew's room and some wool to make Mum a jumper. It was lovely chunky fluffy wool!

Friday 12th April

Today when I woke up, Andrew came into my room and said, "Sally it's a nice day". I got out of bed and the sun was shining. We went barging into Mum's room and said that it was a nice day and could we go to Alton Towers. We pleaded for ages. Finally, she got up and phoned Auntie Janette. She agreed that it was a nice day, so, in a few seconds we were all dressed and ready, so off we went; first to Auntie Janette's and then to Alton Towers. The first thing I went on was the roller coaster; that was brilliant. During the day I went on lots of things such as the Dragon the Octopus and Around the World in 80 Days.

Monday 15th April
Today, at the last minute, I went with the Guides to Drayton Manor Park. I went round with Marianne. I went on the Octopus, the Flying Dutchman, the Waltzers, the Dragon, the log flume and the Para-tower. I had a brilliant time When I got back home I did some ironing for Mum and then watched the snooker on television with the rest of the family.

Saturday 20th April
Today, at 9.00am, I took Robert up to Caroline's house to play with Kathryn. While those two were playing I helped Caroline bath Jonathon. He didn't cry at all. In the afternoon Robert Ellis and Caroline took Kathryn, Robert, and me swimming while Mum looked after Jonathon. At 7.30pm I washed my hair, then, at 8.10pm I watched "The Kenny Everett Show" on television. It was ever so funny as Kenny Everett always is funny.

Sunday 21st April
Andrew's Birthday
Today at 7.00am Andrew woke me up and we went into

Mum's bedroom, and Andrew started opening his presents. He had a dartboard and two sets of darts and a pack of 64 crayons from me. In the afternoon, Uncle Eric and the children came over and Russell Cowdell came for tea as well. We all had a very nice time. At 7.40 pm Mum and me went for a bike ride.

Wednesday 24th April

Mum's birthday

Today I went swimming with class 4 and class 3 had to come too. After swimming it was break time. I had some peanuts. It is Mum's birthday today; she is 36. I bought her a bottle of 'Charlie' perfume and some eye shadow. Mum had a negligee nighty from Dad and a casserole dish from grandma. After school, Catherine Furniss came to play. She stopped for tea and we had a nice time.

Sunday 28th April

Today I went to church and looked after the crèche. Marie helped me. After church we all went out for a meal, which was very nice. After that we went to an antique fair. Dad bought me a little trinket box. It is really lovely and I am going to keep my rings in it.

Monday 20th May
Today, at school, we did spelling and maths. In the afternoon we did our individual topic work. We had a letter to say that May Day had been postponed until June 5th and as I would be on holiday, I was really upset. Anyway, just think, a May Day in JUNE. How utterly stupid!

Wednesday 22nd May
Today, at 6.55am, I woke up and got dressed, because Mum was taking me to Stoke Hospital. When we got there we had to wait for ages, but finally the doctor came and gave me a blood test. Afterwards I went to school for the rest of the day. When I got home I stuck together my gingerbread house. I finished it at 9.30pm and it looked fantastic!

Friday 24th May
Today, as we had a day off school, we went to Hednesford Park for a picnic. We then went to the shopping centre, and I bought a pot of silver nail polish, a little butterfly clip, and a pair of fluorescent socks. In the evening, Mum and me went to see Judy and her new baby girl. She was beautiful.

Sally always enjoyed a bit of 'retail therapy'. She had an eye for a bargain, and used to say that if an item was so cheap it was rude not to buy it!

Wednesday 29th May

Today the weather was beautiful. Robert had the paddling pool out and Andrew and I made an obstacle course. That was fun. In the afternoon, Sarah, Judy and baby Felicity came round. Sarah played with Robert and I had a cuddle with the baby.

Friday 28th June

Today it was the swimming gala. I swam in the front crawl relay; front crawl individual, and back crawl. I won the two front crawling ones and Longdon won the cup with 99 points.

This was Sally's first competitive swimming success, but it would not be her last.

Friday 19th July
End of term

Today I had my grade 1 piano exam; then I went back to school and gave Mrs Beatson a present and a report (for a joke!) In the afternoon it was the end of term service. I played 'Annie's Song' on the flute. When it came to the presentation, I got a cup and a book called 'How to be a cook'. Then Mrs Beatson was presented with a cheque for £60. Mrs Jones was leaving as well; she was presented with a bouquet of flowers. I found it hard to say goodbye to the BEST teacher; Mrs Christine Beatson.

Saturday 27th July
Today, when I woke up, Mum had already gone shopping. In the afternoon I drew some pictures for the little ones in the crèche for tomorrow. When I had finished that, I went into the garden and played cricket with Andrew. I got 54 runs!

Wednesday 7th August
Today I went to my badminton course with Marianne. Afterwards we went for a swim. In the afternoon, Felicity and Sarah Grew came round while Judy went out. When it was time for them to go, Sarah had a paddy and was shouting and crying.

Friday 16th August
Today I finished off my packing and I made the lunch. We had fish fingers and noodle doodles. In the afternoon I played with the Lego and I was just doing the train track, when Marianne came to call. After tea, I had a bath and went to bed, full of excitement about going to Scotland tomorrow morning.

Saturday 17th August
Today, we all got up early and went to Scotland. On the way, I wrote down the names of the products on lorries, and, altogether, got 99. We got to the hotel at 1.30pm and we all jumped in the swimming pool. It was lovely. At 7.30pm we all went for a meal. I had scampi and ice cream.

Tuesday 20th August
Today, Dad went out to play golf and Mum, Robert and me went to the local shop. When we got there the clutch broke on the car and it had to be taken to Aberfoyle Garage. In the evening all the family went to the cocktail party.

Thursday 22nd August
Today, Dad went golfing, Mum did some washing and Andrew had a game of tennis. Before lunch, Mum, Robert, and me went swimming. After lunch, Andrew went down to the canoeing, then Dad, Robert and me went swimming, and Dad jumped in. At 8.00pm, Auntie Barbara and Uncle John came.

Saturday 24th August
Today I woke up at 7.30am and we all went for a swim before breakfast. Then, Dad cooked breakfast and did grilled eggs! It was very funny. Mum, Dad, Andrew and Robert went to Sterling while Auntie Barbara, Uncle John and me went to Aberfoyle. Later we had an hour's indoor bowling.

Sunday 25th August
Today, we all went for a swim before breakfast. Dad dived in twice… he was very good. [Sally was very generous to me as most folks would laugh at my belly flops!] *We all went on a rowing boat, and then we had a game of badminton and then had lunch. In the afternoon, we went to*

Loch Lomond, and the waterfalls were lovely. On the way back, Auntie Barbara, Uncle John, and me climbed part way up a mountain. [John and Barbara are family friends].

Tuesday 27ᵗʰ August
Today, John and Barbara had to go home, but first, we all went for a swim and I did four somersaults in a row. After John and Barbara had gone, we had a game of badminton; then Andrew and I went, on our own, for a meal in the Bonspiel restaurant because Uncle John had given me £10, just for that purpose.

Friday 30ᵗʰ August
Today, Dad and Andrew went golfing while Mum, Robert and me had our usual swim. Dad and Andrew came back about coffee time. Mum and I had a knock at table tennis, and then we went in the solarium for 30 minutes. At 7.00pm we set off for home and arrived at 1.00am, but that did not put me off from writing my diary.

Tuesday 10ᵗʰ December
Today it was school as usual. After school Mum and I had our haircut. At 6.15 we went to the carol concert at Lichfield Cathedral. Lady Diana was there, but we did not see her. When the concert had finished, we rushed outside and saw Lady Diana getting into her Rolls Royce. It was great!

Wednesday 25th December

Today I made a pot of tea and then opened my presents. I had a Panasonic radio cassette, four thimbles, a plug, italic pen, earring case, dressing gown, all-in-one pyjamas, bath hat, hairbrush, cookery book, and a few more things. Andrew had a computer. Andrew bought me two pairs of earrings and a bracelet. I also had two records, shampoo, handbag, £5, trinket box, and a chocolate orange.

Tuesday 31st December
NEW YEAR'S EVE

Today Mum went shopping with Andrew and I played with Robert. In the afternoon I made a piano practise chart. I also watched a bit of 'Gone with the Wind'. At 6.30 'Charlie and the Chocolate Factory' was on TV and it was great. Then Andrew and I stayed up to see the New Year in. It is now 12.21am!

CHAPTER THREE

I'M GOING TO BE A BRIDESMAID!

1986

Sally's 1986 diary was an office business diary with the times of the day marked. Her first entry was as follows:

Wednesday 1ˢᵗ January
8.00 Sleeping
8.30 "
9.00 "
9.30 "
10.00 "
10.30 I got up and had my breakfast.

Monday 13ᵗʰ January
Today it was school. We had morning service, then we did our spellings. We had yucky liver for dinner. In the afternoon I did

a computer graph on cars then, after play, we did some P.E. After school, I had my piano lesson.

Wednesday 22nd January
Today, Mum took me to Stoke Hospital. I had a blood test then; Doctor Tubbs said that I had to have an X-ray. So I had an X-ray. We then went home and on the way we stopped off at an antiques place. I bought a little bug and he is quite cute. Then I went back to school in the afternoon. We did some painting. After school I did some embroidery for a while. At teatime we had pineapple for pudding. Yum Yum.

Wednesday 5th February
We went swimming today. Afterwards we came back to school and read our books. Then we did some maths until playtime. For dinner we had Steak and Kidney Pie. (Yucky!) I did not like it. In the afternoon I had my flute lesson and did some R.E. After school I had my hair trimmed.

Monday 17th February
Beginning of Half Term
I did not get up till quite late this morning. I made a pom-pom for Robert's hats that Mum had made. Mum was making my new curtains. For dinner we had spaghetti on toast (very interesting). In the afternoon I made nine pom-poms. We had curry for tea (Yum Yum) then I had a bath. In

the evening we had a choir practise at our house. I made another pom-pom. Then, Andrew and me had to go to bed – but it was 11.30 pm (Sorry it was 11.10 pm.)

Tuesday 18th February
Today, Mum, Robert, Andrew, and me went to Robert and Nora Edyvean's house. Our Robert stayed with Nora, and Robert (Edyvean) came to Lichfield shopping with us. I went round Tescos with my own trolley and a list. When we got home we had some lunch. Then, I made some more pom-poms in the afternoon. At 8.00pm I watched 'One by One'. It was really good. Then it was time for Andrew and me to go to bed. So that is what we did.

Sally was interested in hospital programmes from an early age, so when the BBC televised a daily edition of 'Hospital Watch' for a week, we recorded each episode for her to watch.

Wednesday 19th February
This morning I watched the morning edition of 'Hospital Watch'. Then I dressed Robert while he was watching 'Postman Pat'. We went up to Castle Ring with some soup and sandwiches for a picnic lunch. We ate them sitting on a tree and I sat half way up for mine. In the evening, I made a large purple, blue, and pink pom-pom. Then, I made a fluffy brown one.

Monday 3rd March
It was school today (boo hoo)
After school, Marie came back to my house, and we went to our piano lessons together. When I got back home, Mum told me that Clare Holland had phoned and said that I could be her BRIDESMAID ON MARCH 22nd.

Wednesday 5th March
I got up early today and Dad took me to Auntie Barbara's. When I got there, Auntie Barbara, Clare, and me went on the bus to Birmingham to fix Clare up with a wedding dress. Ria is going to be the other bridesmaid, and her mum came too. Ria liked trying on the dresses and she was very funny.

Sunday 9th March
Mothering Sunday
The young people's group did the coffee and Marie and I did the crèche. We made little necklaces for the little ones to give to their mums. In the afternoon, I made some scones, nutty chocolate cookies, oatmeal cookies, chocolate brownies shortbread, and some golden crispies. I broke my record by making six items in a day.

Sunday 16th March
This morning we all went to church. Marie and I only had four children in the crèche. After church, we went home and I

sorted out some things that I could bake. After dinner, I made some nutty chocolate cookies, oatmeal cookies, marmalade cake, Bakewell tart, cherry and almond fingers, chocolate caramel squares, and some vanilla slices. I made seven items and broke my record that I had only set last Sunday.

Saturday 22nd March
Clare's Wedding (Mr and Mrs Harle)
Mum and I drove to Dosthill and I had my hair washed and blow-dried. Then I went to Clare's house to put my bridesmaid dress on and so did Ria. A white Rolls Royce took us to the church. After the ceremony LOADS of photographs were taken and then we all went to the reception. After the reception we all went back to Clare's house and some of her friends. Eddie (Clare's brother) *had done Mick's car up. Then Clare and Mick went on their honeymoon. It was a blustery day but it did not spoil their wedding!*

Sunday 30th March
We all went to church and Marie helped me with the crèche. After lunch, Dad set out a treasure hunt, and then Andrew and I went round doing it. Part of the treasure was our Easter eggs and then one clue said that there was some holiday money. We found that and then put together some clues and it spelled 'VILLACANA'. That is where we are going on holiday. It's in Spain. We thought it was GREAT!

Thursday 3rd April

This morning I got up at 7.30 am and at 8.20 am Dad and I went to his office. I worked with Diane all day. I did various things like adding up on the machines and sorting things out. At lunchtime, Dad and I had our sandwiches together. Then we went into town for half an hour. In the afternoon I did more adding up and stuff. Then I was paid my wages of £2 and went home with Dad.

Wednesday 9th April

This morning Dad took me to Tame Valley Alloys where Auntie Barbara and Uncle John work. I helped in the canteen until 3.30 pm. Afterwards we went to see Crispin (the horse). I had a good ride on him and it was fun. Then we went back to Barbara's house for tea. Afterwards we went to Tamworth Cash & Carry to buy stuff for the canteen. Then we went home and I had a bath and went to bed.

Monday 21st April

THE QUEEN'S 60TH BIRTHDAY

At nine o'clock this morning the juniors got on a double decker coach and zoomed off to London. We stopped on the way and had an ice-lolly to celebrate our Andrew's birthday. When we got to London we paraded behind the grenadier guards and sang 'Don't Dilly Dally', 'I'd Like to Teach the

World to Sing', and 'Congratulations' before the Queen came out. When she came out we sang the Queen's birthday song. Sarah Ferguson and Prince Andrew were there and I gave Sarah some daffodils and touched Andrew and Sarah. It was great! We then went to collect our medals, mugs, and packed lunches. We stopped at a motorway service station on the way back and ate our packed lunches. We got home at 9.00 pm and watched the highlights of the day on television and saw Andrew and me. We chatted for a long time and then I just flopped onto the bed after the BEST DAY OF MY LIFE.

Wednesday 23rd April
I went to Bucknall Hospital for a check-up this morning and had my usual blood test. We stopped in Rugeley on the way back and Mum bought me a yellow and white bag for our holiday in Spain. I then went back to school. After school I made a birthday cake for Mum. I made it in the pantry so Mum would not see me but she could smell it!

Thursday 24th April
Mum's Birthday
Judy came round after school to see Mum and stayed for a while. Mum had lots of little presents. I had made her a heart-shaped cake with pink icing.

Saturday 31ˢᵗ May
Holiday to Spain
This morning I woke up at 5.00 am. I got up and got dressed and everybody else got up as well. We got on the road at about 6.00 am ish. We stopped at a motorway service station and Mum fell down some stairs and hurt her ankle badly. A girl looked at it and bandaged it up. When we got to the airport, Mum was put into a wheelchair and two fire brigade men came out (they were first aid trained). They bandaged Mum's ankle up nicely and then, at 10.00 am, we got onto the plane and took off. It was a lovely flight. When we arrived in Spain we had to travel in a hire car on the other side of the road. That was a good experience. When we got to Villacana, I had a swim in the biggest pool and in the evening we had a nice meal.

Sunday 1ˢᵗ June
This morning, after breakfast, we all went to Estepona but it was not very exciting on a Sunday so we went back to the villa. I decided to go swimming in the indoor pool and cut my toe pushing off from the steps. I had my toe bandaged up and am now limping around (the same as Mum). In the evening we all went to the cocktail party and I made new friends with Grace and Andrea. When we got back to the villa we had our evening meal cooked by Dad. It was very nice.

Monday 2ⁿᵈ June

This morning we had a bit of a lie in and, after breakfast, we all went to San Pedro to do a bit of shopping. In the afternoon, Mum had to go to the hospital to have an x-ray on her foot. Andrew and me stayed at Villacana and I went to the reception where I met a Spanish girl called Laura, who worked here, and I helped her deliver some papers. She is very nice indeed. At about 7.15 pm, Mum, Dad, and Robert came back and we had pork chops for tea. (Mum had broken a bone in her foot, but only very slightly.)

Tuesday 3ʳᵈ June

This morning, , Andrew, Robert, and me went to a little shop and bought a ball, a pair of goggles and a lilo to float on in the swimming pool. We spent most of the day around the pool and I went in seven times. In the evening, Mum managed to have a bath with her foot sticking out and then we all went to a barbecue. A girl took a photograph, with my camera, of me, and a waiter called Enrique.

Thursday 5ᵗʰ June

When we woke up this morning, the electricity was not working, so we could not have bacon for breakfast. We spent most of the day by the pool and I had six swims. In the evening we went to the pool bar, and two Spanish ladies were dancing. They both were wearing red dresses. One was red and black and the other red and white.

Saturday 7th June

When we got up this morning we made the beds and packed the suitcases ready for blast-off. Dad took a photograph of me with Laura who gave me a red rose to take back. We got on the plane, at Malaga airport, and flew out at 2.30pm. It took us two hours and forty minutes to get back to Manchester. We collected our luggage and our car and then blasted off home.

Tuesday 10th June

It was meant to be the May Day celebrations at school today, but they had to be cancelled because of the rain. I came third with both my floating bowl and miniature garden. After school, Janette and the children were at home and an animal came into our house. It was a ferret! We had to get a man to catch it and he took it over the stream to the field, but it got back over and came into our house again We managed to get rid of it in the end.

Wednesday 11th June

It was swimming this morning. I did not really want to go so I forgot my pyjamas, accidentally on purpose. During the day our class did English and, in the afternoon, the photographer came. He was the usual funny one. In the evening I watched Top of the Pops and Aha were the highest new entry at number 16 with Hunting High and Low. It is brilliant.

Monday 16th June
It was school today. Yuck! We did not do much in the morning but, in the afternoon our class went to either Lichfield or Rugeley. I went to Lichfield on a town survey. It was quite good fun messing about, because messing about, is mainly what we did.

Sunday 22nd June
This morning we all went to church and Marie and I did the crèche. After lunch, I put on my new blue and white dress and we all went to Carole's garden party in aid of the playgroup. We stayed until the end and I was on a stall. We watched the football on TV in the evening. It was England v Falklands★. Maradona, who played for the Falklands, scored a goal, but he cheated and used his hand to get it in. The Falklands won 2-0. Silly old Maradona!
★ I think that should be Argentina!

Friday 27th June
Our class had Mrs Hudson today for statistics and English. In the afternoon we only messed about. After school, it was hot. So, I put some cold water in our paddling pool and had a dip and a bathe and a dip and a bathe. Dad came home at 6.15pm, driving his new Saab 9000i. The personalised number plate is GRA1V and it stands for _ G = Graham; R = Robert; A = Andrew; 1 = 1st daughter Sally; and V = Valerie. We had a ride in it and it is BRILLIANT!

Friday 18th July

End of primary school for me

This morning we cleared drawers out and did any odd jobs. At dinnertime somebody started off the three cheering business and it went on and on! In the afternoon it was the leavers' service. They did the prize-giving first and I had my cycling certificate and three other things and I also had the leavers' bible. After school we dropped Robert off at Grandmas to stay the night while the rest of us, including John and Barbara, went out for a meal. I had prawn cocktail, fillet steak, and orange and lemon sorbet for sweet. Afterwards we went back to Barbara's for a while and then I got to bed at 12.05 midnight!

Wednesday 23rd July

Royal Wedding (Sarah and Andrew)

I was up early this morning to watch the preparations for the royal wedding. It was lovely. The dress that Sarah wore was ivory and was beautiful. She had four bridesmaids and four pageboys. The youngest pageboy was Prince William, who is only four years old. It was lovely when everybody appeared on the balcony. Princess Diana was holding Prince Harry. Lady Diana was wearing a turquoise dress with black spots and a big sash around her middle. In the afternoon, Mum, Robert, and me went round to Judy's house. We had a little party and I dressed Sarah up as a bride. She looked really sweet. What made everybody laugh was when I showed everyone her blue garter. It was really a blue ribbon.

Sally was always very industrious and hard-working, whether it was cooking, craftwork, swimming, or even logging!

Saturday 9th August
This morning, I got up early and by 8.30 am I was outside getting logs in. Dad said that he would give Andy and me 1 penny a log for holiday money. I had done quite a lot before I went with Dad to the tip with some rubbish. When we got back I did some more logs before going out with Mum for a short while. I did more logs before lunch when I had done just over 400 logs. By 3.00 pm I had done 1000 logs. No, sorry, 1001 logs. I had earned £10 and the log store was really quite full.

Tuesday 2nd September
Started Friary Grange School
I got up and got ready for school this morning. Di Asplin took Marie, Natalie, Abigail and me all together to Friary. We were put into our tutor groups. I was with Marie in classroom S4, and the class was called 1a. We were given our timetable and our tutor's name is Miss Parton. After break we had CDT; it stands for Craft, Design, and Technology.

Then it was dinnertime. I had a Cornish pasty with beans. In the afternoon, we had French and Maths. Then, we went home.

Saturday 6th September
I went into Mum's bed this morning and then I got up. At about 11.15 am Kathryn Ellis came to play with Robert. I made some bath crystals with Kathryn and in the afternoon, we took her to Cannock baths. Kathryn came down the water chute with me about 8 times. SHE LOVED IT. In the evening I watched a drama series called 'Casualty'. Then I went to bed.

Wednesday 10th September
I woke up early this morning and set off to Bucknall Hospital with Mum for my check-up. I had my usual blood test and then went for a walk with Mum. I arrived back at school in time for my history lesson. After school I played shoe shops with Robert and the kitchen man came again.

Saturday 13th September
It was the village show today. I entered mince pies, scones, and decorated fairy cakes. Later on I found out that I had won 1st prize in all three. I won a lovely cookery book and £2.35 in prize money. So, I did quite well really.

Friday 24th October
I went with Dad to the office today as Mum had gone to Denman College with Judy. I cooked the tea when we got back home and then put Robert to bed. I watched the 9 o'clock news while Andrew tickled my feet and I tickled his. After the news, Mum phoned to say she was enjoying herself. Andy and I then went to bed.

Wednesday 5th November
At school today we had classical studies and drama. We then had horrible hockey. Gosh, how I hate hockey. After playtime it was horrible history; that was boring. After lunch we had a talk by a police officer about road safety and accidents. After school, I did my homework and then went out to the bonfire behind the club. I had a good time.

Wednesday 24th December
I had a lie in this morning and then, later on, I called at Marie's to practise the music for tomorrow morning in church. After lunch, the carpet fitter came to lay the new carpet in the kitchen. In the evening I watched 'The Two Ronnies' on television. I then had a long chat with the rest of the family, and then I took my stocking upstairs and went to bed.

Thursday 25th December
It was brilliant this morning. For Christmas, Santa (HO

HO HO!) had brought me a flute. I was overjoyed. I also had green ear muffs, wellies, green slippers, a heart-shaped cake tin, a fountain pen, two sets of bobbles, a chocolate selection box, writing paper, music case, needlepoint book, poetry book, body spray, black track suit, three thimbles, a Mission Praise music copy, pot of Copydex, £2, and a Satsuma. I did really quite well. We went to church and then had Christmas dinner. In the afternoon I opened more presents from grandma, Andrew and my friends. I flaked into bed that night because I was very tired. I had a lovely Christmas day.

CHAPTER FOUR

MAYBE THE SAME WILL HAPPEN WITH MY DIARY

❧

1987

Wednesday 28th January
Dad took me to Bucknall Hospital this morning. We waited for ages and then Dr Tubbs was with us for ages. We went home for a coffee and then I went to school. In the evening Dad and I went shopping to Safeway, as Mum was not feeling too well.

Friday 13th February
We had a normal day at school, then, at 7.30 pm, there was a Valentine disco. I went and Duncan gave me a Valentine's card. I danced with him just about all the time. He even gave me a few kisses. We generally had a brilliant time. Dad collected me at 10.00 pm. I told Mum all about it and then went to bed.

Monday 16th February

School was a little bit of a disaster today, because Duncan said that he did not want to go out with me any more. I was a bit upset. After school I was generally cheesed off. I had my piano lesson at 5.30 pm. When I got home I had tea and then did a jigsaw.

Thursday 19th February

At school I had home economics and our group started needlework. We did an experiment in science and I finished off my paintings in art. After school, we all went to the dentist. Later on, Dad told us that he had booked a holiday in Nottingham, in the forest. It sounds BRILLIANT.

Friday 20th February

It was brilliant at school today because, at dinnertime, seven of us girls played Chinese whispers, and it was really funny. Then, a boy in our class showed me a birthday card that he had bought for Duncan. It said 'Be careful, accidents can cause people'. At 6.30 pm I went to a young people's group meeting and when I got back home, we all played cards.

Monday 30th March

We had our usual day at school and it was as boring as ever. After school, a lady came to our house who had a diary that belonged to a lady who used to live in our house. It was a

great discovery and was fun to look at. I hope (maybe) the
same will happen with my diary.

If ever I needed encouragement to write Sally's story, with the help of her diaries, it was that last sentence. The diary she mentions, found in the drawer of a piece of furniture sold at auction, was written by Margaret Jane Seddon between 1861 and 1864. Margaret was the daughter of Dr Joshua and Mrs Margaret Seddon and lived at 'The Cottage' until she married Frederic Yeld in Longdon church in October 1864.

There were many 'coincidences' (or should that be synchronicities) between Sally and Margaret; they both kept a daily diary, shared the same second Christian name, and attended Longdon church, where they were both married.

Sunday 26th April
It was Robert Ellis's last ever service at St. James and it was
very sad.

Sunday 3rd May
At church this morning we had a doddery old vicar; I did the
crèche.

Sunday 21st June

The service this morning, we had another old fogey, but, in the afternoon, Mum and I helped prepare for the induction of the new vicar, Peter Holliday. We went in the evening to the service. The new vicar has three children; Hellen, who is 13, James, who is 10, and Juliette, who is 3. They are a very nice family and it was a very enjoyable evening.

Friday 26th June

Mum and I went shopping and did various boring things. In the evening, at 9.00 pm, we went to see Ken Dodd at the Civic Hall. Gosh, he is very, very, funny. We had a really good old laugh.

Sally had been unwell for several days and was due for another visit to Bucknall Hospital.

Wednesday 1st July

Mum took me to Bucknall this morning. Dr Tubbs said that I COULD NOT have my TB injection. I somehow found that exceedingly funny! I had my blood test and even had my blood pressure taken.

Wednesday 8th July

I enjoyed tennis today. History was very boring (what a surprise!). Just before our French lesson, Mum collected me and took me to Stafford Hospital for a blood test because, apparently, my platelets are low, whatever they are. On the way home, we stopped at Rugeley and Mum bought me a groovy bikini.

Wednesday 12th August
Dad took me to Bucknall this morning. I had a blood test, and then Dr Tubbs said that I would have to have another barium meal. He said that you have to drink some yoghurt. I mean, really, it tastes more like grit. Yuck! When we got back home we went swimming to join Mum in the pool.

Friday 14th August
At 8.45 am, the tree men came to take down one of our massive lime trees. It is about twice the height of our house. Anyway, they had this equipment that goes really high. Andrew and I had a ride in it. At the end of the day, all the wood had been taken away and you would not have known that it had been up in the morning. It was an amazing day and very interesting.

Saturday 15th August
Mum and Dad's anniversary
I had made a cake for the anniversary. It was a mint and chocolate marble heart cake with mint chocolate on the top. Also, Andrew and I had made some peppermint creams, spelling out 'Happy Anniversary'. There was excitement later

on when Dad found a family of mice – 5 babies and mother. The babies were only very, very tiny – they were beautiful. Also we found a newt. Yuck! At 6.45 pm we went to see 'Superman 4' at The Plaza in Rugeley. It was really good.

Friday 28th August
I finished Anna's birthday cake this morning. Later on we went over to Anna's and had some lunch. We came away just as her party was starting. At 5.00 pm Neil Hoskison [Sally's friend, Marianne's dad] collected me and we popped off to Wales. We got there at 9.30 pm and I camped with Maz.

Saturday 29th August
When I woke up it was raining very hard and we had to stay in the caravan until it stopped. Then, at 2.00 pm, Marianne, Katy and Me went on a pony trek. We set off back home at 4.00 pm and had a good old gas in the car. We talked about what names we would call our children if we have any. I decided on Alicia Jane for a girl, and Francis something for a boy. We got home at 8.30 ish and I had lots of stories to tell Mum and dad.

Saturday 5th September
It was the sponsored bike ride today. The vicar drove us all, plus the bikes in a trailer, to Draycott. We then worked our way back, calling at different churches. Marianne's pedal went

totally duff at Kings Bromley but, luckily, we bumped into Neil, who phoned Maggie, to bring out another bike. When we got back home, Mum and I had a facemask on and went down to Andrew, who was engrossed in watching TV, and we scared him to death. Mum and I found it really, really, funny.

Saturday 26th September
I went to Marianne's birthday party. We played badminton and had a swim. When I got home, I tarted Mum up because they are going to a Tramps and Tarts Ball. Mum looked very tarty by the time I had finished with her. Then, Dad got himself done up as a tramp. He hasn't shaved for two days so his face is really rough, and he put soot on his face as well. I messed his hair up for him. Then, at about 8.30 pm, Carole and Jason Ellis, and Caroline and Robert Ellis [no relation] arrived. Robert had not got dressed up but all the others looked really great. Jason had blacked out his teeth and looked one heck of a mess. It was really funny.

Thursday 1st October
Mum took me to Bucknall this morning. I then went to the City General Hospital for a barium meal (super disgusting). I saw this yucky stuff travelling down my insides. It was quite groovy to watch. We came home and I went to bed because I did not feel too good, but I was feeling better later.

Sunday 4th October

It was the Harvest Service this morning and I did the reading. In the afternoon, the lady who found the very interesting Victorian diary came with her husband, and had a good chat with Mum and Dad.

Tuesday 27th October

Mum took Maz, Andy and me to Walsall today and bought me a mauve jumper, purple material for a blouse, and some other material for a skirt. They are all beautiful. When we got back home, Dr Tubbs phoned to say that I will have to have a bone marrow test, and it will involve a small general anaesthetic. YUCK. I am really upset about that because I don't want to have it.

Sunday 15th November

At church today, Mum and Dad were confirmed by the Bishop of Wolverhampton. In the afternoon a photographer came to do a story about the Victorian diary of Jane Seddon, and wanted to take some photographs of me. I think he took about 60!!

Tuesday 24th November

This afternoon we went by coach to London to the Royal Albert Hall and saw the school's prom. It was fantastic. I saw the man who hosts 'Blockbusters' (Bob Whateverhisnameis), and Richard Stilgoe, the poet. It was a fantastic evening. We got home at 1.45 am and I got to bed at about 2.15 am.

Monday 30th November
I had to go to Stoke General Hospital for a bone-marrow test. I was supposed to have a general anaesthetic but, instead, I had gas. It was rather a doss, but, when I came to my senses, my back hurt where they had taken the bone marrow. I hobbled around for the rest of the day like an old granny!!

Thursday 17th December
I went to school until break-time, when Dad collected me and off we went to Bucknall Hospital. I had a blood test and it hurt a lot today. Dr Tubbs told us that I had a swollen oesophagus, and the veins could burst and, if they do, I will need a blood transfusion. He also told us that I would, almost certainly, need a new liver at some stage in my life. He said it could be in 5, 10, 15, 20, or 25 years' time – he is just not certain. I was upset to hear this news, but I have now just about got over it.

That night was the first time that Val had seen me cry; sadly it would not be the last. It was around the time that little Ben Hardwick was in the news. He was suffering from a failing liver and, sadly, died after undergoing a liver transplant. He was the first child to receive a liver transplant.

Thursday 31st December

Mum took me down to Lichfield to have my hair cut quite short. I then had it Scrunched dried, so now it looks as if it is permed. In the afternoon, Angela, Helen and family came and stayed the night. We saw the New Year in and then went to bed at about 12.30am HAPPY NEW YEAR EVERYONE AND GOOD MORNING

CHAPTER FIVE

THE DOGS

❧

1988

Friday 5th February
I went to school with my uniform on back to front and a red
nose on today. We had a great laugh at school. After school I
mainly watched telly all evening because it was COMIC
RELIEF. At about 11.00 pm I phoned in myself and we
pledged £10; it was great! I was laughing all evening, it was
really great, and when we think about it our £10 could get
20 children immunised against 6 fatal diseases and I think
that's great!

Is this the first indication of her vocation as a nurse?

Saturday 19th March
Mum, Andrew, Robert and me went to Lichfield. I transferred
my 'piggy' account to 'on line' and I have got a really groovy
folder with a calculator. We also went into 'The Kitchen

Shop' where there was a chocolate moulding demonstration going on. We bought some chocolate and some moulds. After dinner I started having a go with the chocolate moulding, and then Andrew came in and said could I get some food for two collie dogs that were in our kennel. So I did and went outside to see them. They were really cute but are very thin and it is a mystery where they have come from.

Sunday 20th March
At 7.00 am I got up and dressed this morning. I went out to see the dogs; they were still there!

We all went to church. After our lunch we took the two dogs to Rugeley police station. I was quite sad. I made some more chocolates; they were lemon creams. I did not do much in the evening except for the fact I was in a silly giggly mood.

When we took the dogs to the police station I knew we shouldn't have said 'let us know what happens to them'. Two weeks later we received a call to say no one had claimed them and they were going to be put down. Did we want them? We ended up buying them back!

Our first dog Sadie had died at 3 years old with a tumour. We had always intended having another dog but had been otherwise occupied with three children, and a stray cat that we had took in.

Monday 11th April

I had my piano lesson at 10.00 am. I enjoyed it. Then Mum and I went into town and bought two dog leads. After some cheese rolls for dinner, Andrew, Mum and me went to fetch the dogs. They were really excited, and when we got home, half the village was round to look at them. Later on, after tea, Dad, Andrew and me took them to the vets. They were very good. We have named the male SAM and the female LUCKY.

Thursday 23rd June

I shan't tell you anything about school because it was boring and also because at 6.00 pm I went to school ready to perform in 'Oliver' at 7.30 pm. It was great, I really enjoyed it. Grandma and Granddad came to watch it and Mum came. Afterwards, we took Grandma and Granddad home. Lucky came with us because she had been on stage! (Playing the part of Bullseye). Everything was great!

Thursday 14th July

I had my piano exam today. The examiner was a lady. That was a change! Before we went to the exam we took Lucky to the vet to be spayed. We fetched her at 5.00 pm. She was all weak and shivery so she slept for a lot of the time and I am going to sleep in the kitchen with her tonight.

Friday 15th July

I didn't go to school today because I had a slightly disturbed night with the dogs and also I had to look after the dogs because Mum had to take Andrew to the hospital about his finger. He had fractured it slightly. In the afternoon Mum went to a do at Dad's office and I made a lemon cake and some biscuits. The dogs are sleeping together in the kitchen again tonight. Lucky is recovering well.

Thursday 21st July

School was great today because we did hardly any work. After lunch we had 'Crackerjack'; presented by Mr Martin and Miss Parton. Mrs. Craig, Mr. Atkin, and Mr. Page took part and they all got 'gunged'. It was really funny. After school I bathed Sam.

Wednesday 27th July

Before whizzing off to Derbyshire, Andrew had to go to the dentist.

When we got to Ashbourne, we had lunch, and then walked up the Tissington Trail. After walking so far, Mum and Andrew walked back to get the car while Granddad and me walked on and met them in the next car park. We then went in the car to Hartington Youth Hostel. After making our own tea we phoned Dad and then grandma. Grandma had bad news that Auntie Mary had died. We had a game of cards and then showered and went to bed. Mum and I are in Dormitory 1.

Saturday 30th July
We all walked along the Tissington Trail to Biggin and then caught a bus back to Hartington. We came home and Dad had cooked the tea. I am glad we are home because I was beginning to miss Dad and my beautiful dogs.

Monday 1st August
I didn't do much today or it didn't feel as if I did. I cleaned out the kennel and the rest of the morning ticked by. At 2 o'clock I went off with Marianne for a game of badminton. When I got back home, Mum's Aunt Enid and cousin, Maureen had called in and we had a nice chat. Later I nearly dozed off, because I was cuddling Lucky and she was fast asleep.

Thursday 4th August
Mum and I set off early to pick up Grandma and Granddad and then off to Auntie Mary's funeral in Whittlesea, near Peterborough. It was very sad. I met a few more of the family afterwards. We got back home at 7 o'clock.

Saturday 6th August
We got up at 4.00 am and were on the road, heading for Scotland, at 4.40 am. We travelled 420 miles to Lochanully.

We are staying in a little wooden chalet and I am sharing a room with Robert. It hasn't got a dressing table so all my cosmetics are on a chair! We had our tea in the chalet and then went for a swim in the small indoor pool.

Monday 8th August
We went to Nairn today and the beach was lovely. We had a quick look round the town and went into a needlework shop and the lady there knew Susan Ryder [Our neighbour.] I had a little swim in the sea. I was a bit scared of any jellyfish, but I was OK. The Duchess of York has had her first baby today and it is a girl.

Friday 12th August
We went off to the Cairngorm Mountains and went in the chairlift to the top. It was ace! We got back to the chalet for lunch, which we had on the patio. The lads went off to play golf whilst Mum and I had a game of snooker! I won on the black!! In the evening we had a meal out and were served by Mum's favourite waiter, whose name is Martin.

Friday 19th August
We set off home at 6.00 pm, after our week at Forest Hills, and arrived at 1.30 am. The dogs are fine and were pleased to see us.

Thursday 25th August
I was first up (apart from Dad). I walked the dogs and then had a cooking morning. At 2 o'clock Mum went to see Wendy Tydeman, who has just had an operation, and I went to Sue Ryder's house for three hours. When I got home, nobody was in, so I got the dogs out of the kennel, and they sat in the kitchen with me, whilst I did my embroidery.

In September Sally returned to school as a third year but, from her diary entries, was not finding school stimulating and hospital visits were continuing to interrupt her studies. She was enjoying practical things such as cooking, babysitting for friends and needlework assignments, which she did for Sue Ryder's business. There were also mentions of practices for the annual church harvest supper concert. She was keeping fit with cycling, walking and swimming.

Thursday 8th September
I had to go to Stafford Hospital to see Doctor Gibson. I asked him if he would sponsor me for the cycle ride, and he did. I went to school in the afternoon and had French and Geography. After school, I finished my Brackley Town Hall [needlepoint picture] *and took it to Sue's and got £7 for it. It was my turn to wash up the dinner pots, and after that I did my homework.*

Saturday 10th September

I took my produce show exhibits to the village hall and then set off with Dad on the sponsored cycle ride. We started at Handsacre Church and Mum, Andrew and Mary Pratt joined us later. We managed to visit 10 churches in 20 miles. It was great but I was tired in the evening.

Sunday 11th September

We all went to church for family service. Carole sang the song she had composed; it was lovely. After the service I collected some of my sponsor money. I don't know what was the matter with me, but I felt a bit down so, later on I went on my bike to see Carole for a lovely chat.

Saturday 8th October

The harvest supper concert went really well. Dad had a custard pie in his face, which was rather funny.

Sunday 23rd October

After lunch, Auntie Rosie, Uncle Ray, James, And Olivia came but, just as they arrived, Mum and Dad were returning from walking the dogs when they ran off and were missing for two hours. Dad, Ray, and Jason Ellis went looking for them, and, eventually they came back on their own! Typical!

Tuesday 25th October
We went to Drayton Manor Park today; poor old Dad had to go to work. Carole and the children came and also Andrew's friend, Robert Hickinbottom (Hicky). We had a great day and the weather was fine. I went on just about everything.

Wednesday 2nd November
Back to school.
I didn't enjoy the thought of going back to school today but it wasn't too bad. After school, I had a letter from the hospital to say that I have got to have a liver biopsy on the 12th December at the Queen Elizabeth Hospital in Birmingham, so I am very cross.

Monday 12th December
Mum and Dad brought me into hospital this morning. Mum stayed with me and Dad went off to work. A lady doctor came to see me in the afternoon and had a prod at my tummy, but I didn't see Doctor Elias. Uncle Peter came in at 5.30 pm and took Mum home at 6.00 pm. I phoned Dad and, after tea, phoned Andrew to say I probably wouldn't be out until Friday.

Tuesday 13th December

I didn't have a very good night's sleep and a fire alarm woke us up at 6.00 am. I had a blood test at 8.30 am and Mum arrived at 10.00 am. A little later on I had an injection and then a liver scan. I felt really faint after the injection. In the afternoon the lady doctor gave me an injection of vitamin K, which took ages. At 6.30 pm Dad, Andrew and Robert came to see me. After they had gone I phoned Peter Holliday and had a lovely long chat. Later on I phoned Marie and she may be coming to see me.

The following day's entry was written in a bit of a scrawl with the explanation that it was written left-handed as 'my thing for putting drips into me was still in the back of my right hand and IT HURT'.

Wednesday 14th December

I started the day with a blood test and then went down to have my ultrasound scan, which was brilliant. I then had 6 units of platelet drip into the back of my hand, which really hurt. Then I had my biopsy, which was OK. Peter Holliday came to see me and then, just as I was having my tea, Marie and Di arrived and we had a lovely chat. I phoned Grandma later on.

Thursday 15th December
My temperature was fine this morning, so, when the doctors came round they said I could go home. I phoned Mum and Judy brought her in. While I was waiting, a really nice nurse called Ruth took out the amazing contraption in the back of my hand. I am really glad to be home so I can see my mega dogs!

Wednesday 21st December
I went to school today for the last day of term. I had lots of presents, including a rude one from Colin. In the evening we all went to Mrs Grew's house [Douglas's mum] *and had a good old carol sing and then some supper. I really enjoyed it.*

Thursday 22nd December
I had a nice lie in and then started to ice the Christmas cake. I ran out of icing sugar but Mum was taking Andrew to his friend's house so she called at the shop on the way back. While they were gone, I had a lie down with the dogs on top of me! I finished icing the cake after lunch, and then took Natalie and Marianne their presents. In the evening we all had a game of Scrabble, and I very nearly won.

Friday 23rd December
Mum and I went shopping quite early and, when we got back, I played a few carols on the piano. In the afternoon, we had a

little party and Rebecca, Adam, Judy, Sarah, Felicity, Juliette, and Hellen came. I babysat for Judy later on and, while they were out, wrapped up all her presents. It was great fun.

Saturday 24th December
I had a lovely lie in and then took Sam for a walk. Later on we all went to Dad's office to tidy his room and put his new desk in. Mum went off to collect Grandma and Granddad and we came home with Dad. I went to bed at a reasonable time, all excited at the thought of tomorrow.

Sunday 25th December
I had lots of presents from Santa, including a typewriter and track suit. In the afternoon we opened the presents under the tree. I had bought Mum and Dad Pictionary and later on we all had a game. It was quite late when I got to bed.

Monday 26th December
I didn't get up until 10.00 am and then Granddad and I took the dogs for a walk on Cannock Chase, while everyone else, except Grandma, went for a bike ride. Later on, I wrote a letter, on my new typewriter, to Uncle Cyril [Sally's great uncle, who she regularly wrote to after his wife died].

Tuesday 27th December

I took both of the dogs for a walk this morning, and they were fine, mainly because we didn't see any other dogs! We then took Grandma and Granddad home and went for lunch at Uncle Peter and Auntie Joan's.

Friday 30th December

Dad went back to the office today. Halfway through the morning, Mum was worn out so we made her lie down and watch 'Back to the Future' on television.

Saturday 31st December

At 8.00 pm, Carole, Rebecca, and our family went to the Hollidays' for supper and a game of cards. Then, Hellen and I stayed in to look after the little ones while everyone else went to Midnight Mass. At 11.55 pm, Jason and Adam rang the doorbell, which gave Hellen and me a bit of a fright. (Jason hadn't been very well, so that's why he didn't come in the first place). Dad and Ruth collected us after the service and we joined in the party, which was really enjoyable. It is now 2.20 am, so I think I had better get some sleep before I go to church in the morning.

CHAPTER SIX

HAPPY 15TH BIRTHDAY

1989

Sunday 1ˢᵗ January

I woke up at 10.00 am and we all went to church, except Andrew, who is still in bed. After lunch we all went for a lovely walk on Cannock Chase. Dad and I walked back from Upper Longdon while everyone else went in the car. Of course we took the dogs with us and they had a lovely time, taking it in turns to be off the lead. It was lovely to watch them. When we let Sam off he jumped right over Lucky; it was really funny. After tea I fed the dogs and then brushed them to get rid of the mud.

Saturday 14ᵗʰ January

I decided that Andrew and I would go to Sutton Coldfield on the train; so that is exactly what we did. I bought Robert some little cars for his birthday and a scientific calculator and bikini for me. Andrew and I bought a compact disc for Dad's birthday. We got back to Lichfield at 3.00 pm and Mum collected us from the station.

After several days of feeling unwell, Val took Sally to the doctors, who advised going straight to Stafford Hospital, where they kept her in for several days while they carried out tests. One of the tests, which Sally would have to endure many times, was a gastroscopy. This is where a tiny camera is inserted into the gullet, enabling the doctor to inspect the veins in the oesophagus and, if necessary, inject a damaged vein to seal it and prevent it causing a haemorrhage.

Tuesday 24ᵗʰ January
Today I was told that I was to have a gastroscopy. They took me to theatre and put me to sleep and then injected my veins internally. When I came round back on the ward, Peter Holliday was there but I was too sleepy to talk much, and my throat was sore. Mum went home when Dad arrived but came back later to stay the night with me. I had a much better night's sleep.

Wednesday 25ᵗʰ January
Doctor Gibson came to see me and said that I could now have food and drink, so I had a few sips of orange squash. Granddad came in on the bus to see me, and, while he had

gone off to have his lunch, Di Asplin came in and brought me a Minnie Mouse nighty. After Granddad and Di left I rested in the afternoon, and in the evening Ruth and Hellen Holliday and Dad and Robert came to see me.

Friday 27th January

I got up after having a lovely night's sleep and had a wash and spruce up. Doctor Gibson didn't come but sent a message that I would have to stay in for one more day. I played a few games with Mum and Uncle Eric came to see me and later on Sarah George came in. Dad brought Andrew and Robert in later.

Saturday 28th January

Mum popped off to the town, thinking that Doctor Gibson would be in late morning, but he came just after Mum had left and said I could go home. I will need to come back for another internal injection on Tuesday. We got home at midday and I had a good sleep in the afternoon. I woke up at teatime and then had what I had been waiting for; A BATH. It was heaven!

Tuesday 31st January

I had a bit of a lie in but then had to go to Stafford Hospital for my second gastroscopy. A doctor put a Venflon in the back of my right hand (and that is why my writing is weird). It *really hurt, and I don't think he made a very good job of it. Doctor Gibson came to see me at 6.15 pm and said I could go home.*

Friday 10th February
I had another full day at school and quite enjoyed it, apart from the maths test. After school Mum told me that my next gastroscopy would be next Thursday and not Tuesday. So, I have an extra couple of days to worry about it! After tea, Andrew went to a school disco and Dad and I assembled a cabinet for the new midi hi-fi. It looks great, but it did take quite a lot of brainpower.

Tuesday 14th February
Dad had sent Mum and me a joint Valentine card saying:
Roses are red,
Carnations are pink,
This card may not be from whom you think.
I have to confess, there are two girls in my life,
One is my daughter, the other is my wife!!
Mum and Dad went out to their Bishop's Certificate course in the evening. I shall now try to get to sleep, even with two dogs on my bed!!

Thursday 16th February
I went to school first thing for my chemistry test, and then

Mum collected me to go to Stafford Hospital again for another gastroscopy. Doctor Gibson came to see me afterwards and I asked him about my liver biopsy. He said that they had taken muscle instead of liver – so they have made a real mess of that! Fortunately, I don't have to have another one.

Wednesday 22nd February

I was up early this morning and went with Dad to his office. Then, at 9.30 am, he took me to Tamworth railway station where I met Granddad. We got on a train to Nuneaton, changed for Peterborough, and then caught a bus to Whittlesey. Uncle Cyril met us and we went back to his flat for lunch. After looking at photographs and chatting we walked round to Heather's house (Cyril's daughter) where we saw baby Ashley. He is lovely, and only five weeks old. I am staying the night at Heather's and Ashley has just had his late feed.

Tuesday 7th March

I was in a good mood this morning, so instead of saying things, I sang them! I had a fit of the giggles in English. The royal helicopter landed on the playground, as they were practising for when the Queen Mother comes.

Monday 13th March

We got our assessments at school today; mine wasn't too bad.

After tea I went to baby-sit at Judy's. I watched 'Panorama'.
It was about the health service and how the government are
going to put a limit on how much the health service can
spend. I am against this particular budget.

Thursday 16th March
I can't have any breakfast this morning as Mum is taking
me to Stafford for another gastroscopy. I had to wait around
for ages before being taken down to theatre. I didn't have a
Venflon this time, just a little butterfly needle in the back of
my hand. I have to stay in overnight as there was a slight
problem with the injections. Mum went home at about 6.30
pm and Dad is coming in later. Whilst Dad was still with
me, they moved me to a different ward with other ladies; so
I hope they don't snore, otherwise I shan't get much sleep!
Friday 17th March
I woke up at 6.00 am because the lights all went on, and I
didn't really doze off again. Doctor Gibson came to see me
at about 7.15 am and said I could go home. I asked him if
it was possible to have some teeth out in preparation for my
brace, when I have my next gastroscopy. He said he would
arrange it.

Saturday 1st April
All Fools Day!
Andrew and I played a really good trick on Mum and Dad;

we put the clocks forward an hour and they didn't notice for ages. Dad went to get some cement from a shop at what he thought was 9.25 am but was really 8.25 am, and I am surprised the shop was actually open! We had lunch in the garden, and then I sunbathed and read my book for a while. Rob, Juliet, Simon, and Mark Heaton came for dinner. We had a lovely evening, and the baby (Mark) is lovely. He is really sweet and bouncy. They went home at 10.30 pm after a really good game of cards.

Tuesday 18th April
School was brilliant today because at midday the big red royal helicopter landed and the Queen Mother was in it. She was really sweet and ever so small! I really enjoyed games in the afternoon. We played rounders and tennis.

Thursday 20th April
I got up and fed and walked the dogs as I can't have any breakfast today. We set off to Stafford at 10.00 am for another gastroscopy. I was less than an hour in theatre and came home at 6.30 pm. I had a few chicken nuggets!

Friday 21st April
Andrew had a lovely birthday and had a tennis racquet, badminton racquet, and six tennis balls, and lots of other bits

and pieces. I had the day off school, as I wasn't feeling 100%. I stayed in bed for most of the morning, and then I went for a little walk and bought Andrew some chocolate as a little extra present.

Saturday 22nd April

We are all going to Wychnor Park today and are staying the night. I prepared the meal for Andrew, Robert and me and Mum and Dad are going to the hotel for a meal with Carole, Jason, Judy, Douglas, Peter, and Ruth. At about 11.00 pm they all came back for a game of cards. Judy had made a birthday cake for Mum with 40 candles on it! They are being rather noisy, so I don't know if I will get much sleep tonight.

Wednesday 17th May

I went into school first thing and, at break-time, Mum collected me and took me to Stafford Hospital. I had a blood test and then I saw the orthodontist (Dr Muir). He was really nice. He said that when I have my next gastroscopy he would take four teeth out and a couple of weeks later, he would fix my brace. I went back to school afterwards but after school I felt totally drained, so I had a relaxing evening.

Saturday 20th May

We all got up at 12.15 am and drove to Gatwick for a flight to Malaga. It was a Boeing 727 and it was a brilliant flight.

We were flying at over 500 mph, and one of the male stewards was rather dishy so, of course, that made the flight better. We arrived at Villacana at 12.30 pm and I spent most of the afternoon sunbathing and swimming.

Wednesday 24th May

We did a spot of shopping in the village over the road and then sunbathed by the pool. I played in the pool with Katie, who is 12, and her brother, Kevin, who is 15. Kevin is really nice, and he likes me! Andrew and Dad won a tennis tournament and won a bottle of champagne.

Sunday 4th June

It was family service at church today and there weren't many people there. After lunch, we went to see little Timothy Robert (Robert and Caroline's baby). He is beautiful. I took him the rainbow embroidery I had done in a little red frame.

Saturday 10th June

Dad brought the post up to me in bed. I had a letter from Kevin, so I have read it over and over again. After I had done the ironing for Mum, I wrote a letter back to Kevin (no time like the present!!)

Thursday 15th June

I got up and washed my hair and then at 10.15 am Mum took me to Stafford Hospital for my gastroscopy and teeth out. When the anaesthetist came to see me she said that I didn't have to have a really painful premed injection in my leg, so I am really pleased. When I woke up my mouth felt pretty yuck and I came back to the ward and had a sleep. I later found out that I had to stay the night.

Friday 16th June
I was woken up at 6.00 am to have my temperature and blood pressure taken and, of course, I couldn't get back to sleep again. I got dressed and Dr Gibson came to see me at 7.40 am. He said that he hadn't had to inject any veins in my oesophagus, which was good. Mum collected me at 11.00am and I went into school for the rest of the day. I am really tired now.

Wednesday 19th July
School was quite a laugh today. Mum collected me at lunchtime as I had an appointment at Stafford Hospital to have separators in my teeth. They are just like mini elastic bands, and you can't see them at all, but they feel really weird. I have lots of homework to do tonight.

Saturday 22nd July
We all went to Lichfield and I went to the optician's. It was my favourite optician whose name is Martin. He is really tall and nice, so I love having my eyes tested! He put some contact

lenses in and I walked round the town for 40 minutes. They were fine so I have ordered some. We had rather a silly evening looking at old photos of Andrew, Robert and me as babies. They are really funny.

Sunday 23rd July

We walked up to church this morning and Maureen Lucas asked me if I would be a bridesmaid for her daughter, Liz. I accepted and am really chuffed. The wedding isn't until next July, so I have got time to get to know Liz better.

Monday 24th July

I got up early today and went on the school coach to Derbyshire. We walked by the river Dove; it was beautiful and the weather was hot again. All the teachers had their shorts on; it was really funny. In the evening I cycled up to see Liz Lucas and had a nice chat with her and Maureen.

Tuesday 25th July

I went to school early again today and we went to Ashbourne and got on the Tissington Trail. We hired bikes and sped along the trail really fast; it was great fun. When I got home I went to Sue's until 6.00 pm. At 9.00 pm, Judy collected me and we went up to church to try and trace a map from a slide projection, but it didn't work, so we are going to have to think it out again!

Wednesday 26th July
I had a lie in this morning. I was meant to be going to Derbyshire again but I have to have my brace put in. It wasn't too bad, but it feels weird and I look like Jaws! I went to help with Sarah's birthday party afterwards.

Thursday 14th September
I had no breakfast today as I am going in for another gastroscopy. I walked Sam so I didn't have to smell any toast or see anyone eating breakfast! We went off to Stafford at 10.20 am and I had to wait around until I was taken to theatre at 1 30 pm. It was OK though as Dr Gibson didn't have to inject internally. Just when I was coming round, Carole and Adam came in and whilst they were there I had a blood test. Maureen and Liz came in later on a brought me a beautiful basket of flowers.

Saturday 16th September
Dad and I went off to Safeway's this morning. We both had a trolley and a token for £3 off £30, so we both estimated how much we had spent. I spent £30.28 in my trolley. Close aye! Dad spent about £31.66.

Friday 22nd September
Harvest Supper
School was a bit boring today. After school I had a list of

things to do to prepare for the harvest supper. I sat on a table with Maureen and Vic, Flo, Liz and Colin, and Liz's brother, Stephen and his wife, Caroline. At 9.15 pm the entertainment started and it was great. We had Status Quo, me as Victoria Wood, and Dad and Carole as Kenny Rogers and Dolly Parton. It was really funny. We got to bed at midnight.

Saturday 23rd September
Andrew and Dad went off to the Belfry to watch the Ryder Cup, Robert went to play with Adam, and Mum and I went off to Sutton Coldfield to do some shopping. At 5.45 pm, Alex and Anna came to stay the night as Eric and Janette are going to a party.

Wednesday 27th September
I have decided to join the Friary Singers because Tim has joined, and because I like singing!! Andrew broke the light switch in the bathroom last night, so I had a bath by candlelight tonight.

On the next page was the following note: 'Plan ahead. Buy your 1990 diary now'. Sally had written, 'NO!'

Thursday 28th September
Tim sat behind me in maths today. The bad news is that he

is going out with someone else. We watched a film in biology, which showed an operation of removing a cancerous lung. It was disgusting. After school I went to Sue's. She is paying us differently, so it works out that I will get more (probably because I work faster).

Thursday 5th October
School was a laugh today, especially geography. I just seemed to laugh for the whole lesson and then, in biology, my stool had disappeared, so I pinched Neil's. He then sat down on the floor, it was really funny. After tea, I walked the dogs with Andrew, and Sam bit me. I was really cross with him.

Saturday 7th October
My 15th Birthday
I had a super day today. I had loads of presents. At 9.50, Interflora brought a mini flower arrangement from Maureen and a hat with dried flowers from Liz and Colin. At 10.00 am Maureen came and gave me a 'teddy', which is a pink piece of underwear (like a camisole and French knickers joined together). After an early tea we all went off to Walsall illuminations with Judy and family, Carole and family, and Hellen and Juliette. There was a laser show on a moving screen and it said 'HAPPY 15th BIRTHDAY TO SALLY PASSEY'. It was brilliant.

Thursday 19th October

It's official; Tim is no longer going out with Tara! (Good) On the way home on the bus, Simon sat on my knee. He is a right laugh, but he squashed my knee! (He is a 5th year, and quite nice!)

Sunday 22nd October

I was late up this morning, which wasn't surprising as I went to bed late last night. We managed to get to church on time. It was a really wet morning but I walked Sam after church as he hadn't had a walk this morning. After lunch I did some of my Suffolk embroidery. We had a pleasant day in and I had a giggling fit before and during tea. I just love laughing sometimes.

Wednesday 25th October

I was up slightly later today, but I still walked the dogs. Marianne came round and we went off to play squash. We were a bit early so we watched Simon playing (who sat on my knee the other day). I think that he is rather bosting. He watched us while we played and even lent me his racquet.

Thursday 26th October

I had a relaxing day helping Mum and in the afternoon we made two nightshirts; one for me and one for Sarah. They are pink and white striped with a rabbit on the front. Sarah doesn't know about it yet, so it will be a surprise tomorrow night as we are all going to Center Parks for the weekend. I can't wait until tomorrow.

Mum wrote my diary over the following few days, so I have copied what she wrote.

Friday 27th October
We set off for Center Parks at 10.00 am. We arrived at 11.20 am and booked a few things and waited for the others. Peter and Ruth and family arrived and we went into the dome and had a great time going down the water chutes. Judy and Douglas and Carole and Jason and all the children came and we all had lunch. I went down the rapids, but when I came back I felt terrible and was sick. An ambulance took me to Mansfield Hospital and lots of doctors prodded my tummy and put me on a drip. Mum stayed with me and we had a room to ourselves. I hardly slept at all.

Saturday 28th October
I still have a terrible pain this morning and keep fainting. In the afternoon, Dad came and Mum went off to do some shopping. She bought me some slippers and a book, but I was too weak to be interested in them. I told Mum how much I loved her. They moved me to another ward and then I don't remember what happened. I was taken to theatre and Dr

Fairbrother operated on me and took out my spleen. When I came round I was in intensive care. Mum and Dad stayed all night. Peter came and said that everyone was thinking and praying for me.

October 1989 – Mansfield Hospital

In October 1989 we all went to Center Parks Amusement Park in Nottingham for a long weekend with the families of three very close friends. Little did we realise how long the weekend would turn out to be.

The day we arrived Sally suddenly became very ill after swimming in the indoor pool. She was rushed by ambulance to Mansfield General Hospital. When we told the nursing staff that Sally suffered from a strain of hepatitis they insisted that everyone around the bed must wear protective masks, despite my protestations that her condition was not contagious.

We were desperately worried as it became clear how very poorly she was. I was also very frustrated that they would not contact her consultant in Stafford to obtain essential background on her condition. They decided that she was suffering internal bleeding and so operated late at night to remove her spleen. The surgical team had great difficulty in stemming the bleeding and had to re-operate to finally stop the bleeding. It was the Saturday night when the clocks went back an hour so it was undoubtedly the longest night of our entire lives.

Sally was eventually transferred to intensive care. I remember going for a very early morning walk with Val and steeling ourselves to the unimaginable possibility of losing our precious daughter.

The hospital provided us with a mattress so that we could sleep over in the day room for several nights while Sally fought her first battle for life in intensive care. We were blessed that the surgeon, Mr Fairbrother, was not only at the top of his game but was also a thoroughly nice bloke. Through his skill, the care of the nurses and Sally's fighting spirit, she pulled through and returned home after ten days.

Sunday 29th October
I was nursed by Sandra. I dozed off between doctors and nurses tending to my drips and things. The clocks went back at 3.00 am to 2.00 am and I am having a lot of blood because I am losing more inside. The surgeons are standing by in case I need another operation. I am having more plasma, everywhere hurts, and my nose itches. I want to lie on my side but am not allowed to. I need to sleep; Mum and Dad keep going out of the room. At this stage, Mum and Dad are distraught. They wait in a nearby waiting room with

a pillow and sleeping bag. Mum does yoga exercises, which helps her to keep calm. Doctors, nurses, and the anaesthetist are dashing about for more blood and plasma. At 6.00 am I go to theatre again and the surgeon, Dr Fairbrother, is saving my life. He and his team have been up all night with me. They and Dad all need a shave! Mum and Dad walk hopelessly into the fresh air of the dawn, praying for their precious daughter's life.

At 8.30 am I am brought back to the ward. Mum is anxious to see Andrew and Robert. Nurse Sheila takes over from Sandra. I am hot and very sleepy. Dr Fairbrother tells me that he has taken out my spleen. Andrew, Robert, and Judy come to see me for a few minutes. The chaplain comes to give me communion, but I am asleep, so he gives a small service for the family, Peter and Judy. I have 'get well' letters from all the children, but I am too ill to know yet. I sleep on and off all day with drips, plasma and blood tests, but my tummy is not bleeding. I have a tube in my side to drain off fluid, one up my nose, one under my clavicle, and a catheter to drain my bladder. Mr Vernon is my anaesthetist. He reminded Dad of Blackadder.

Monday 30th October
Mum comes into my room in her red dressing gown. I can't remember Andrew, Robert, and Judy coming to see me. At 9.30 am, Mum helps Bev to bed bath me and they sit me

up a bit. I am still using oxygen to help me breathe. At 10.00 am, Peter came with lovely cold hands to cool me down. Andrew stayed with me a while and talked to me. Robert came in and said he was worried about my drip needles being taken out I told him not to worry. Carole came in as well. At 2.00 pm I was moved onto a ladies' ward. Lovely Nurse Bev has taken over and she has been explaining lots of things to Mum. Mum spends ages brushing my hair. My lips are swollen and dry, but I sleep and sleep. Maureen and Uncle Eric have phoned and send their love. I sleep all night and am doing well. The Sister fixes Mum and Dad to sleep in the day room; the ladies on the ward have a good laugh about Dad sleeping there.

Tuesday 31st October

I feel a bit better this morning. In the night, I asked Mum to sit with me for a while and we had a little chat about God helping to heal me, and all the others in this hospital. A nurse took out the tube from my nose, and that feels great. At 11.30 am they took me in a special chair to the bathroom and lowered me into the water. It was heaven. They took off the dressing and I saw the wound for the first time. After the bath I put on my new nightie and Rev Marriot (congregational minister from my old church) came to see me. A girl called Claire spent some time talking to me.

Wednesday 1ˢᵗ November

I was awake a lot in the night and chatted to Mum for a while. I am looking forward to my bath, but first I have to have the catheter and one of the drains out. Mum stayed with me, and it wasn't as bad as I thought it would be. Peter and Ruth came in and it was lovely to see them but I was feeling exhausted. They came back after lunch and brought me a lovely grey mouse and some flowers. Mum hooked the mouse onto the curtain, so he has a ride every time they are closed.

Thursday 2ⁿᵈ November

Dr Fairbrother said my intravenous drip could come out today. That is good news but I still feel exhausted. Glenys Beveridge [a near neighbour] *phoned to wish me well. Judy and Carole came to see me and, later on, Grandma and Granddad came. It was lovely to see them. They had come on the train to Nottingham and then on a bus to Mansfield. At 6.00 pm, Dad came in with Andrew. Andrew and Mum went off to McDonalds and brought Dad a Big Mac back. Dad went off into the day room to eat it. I didn't get much sleep and I want to go home.*

Friday 3ʳᵈ November

Dr Fairbrother said I was doing really well and I might be able to go home on Sunday. Mum asked if she could take a photo of him and the bald American doctor, David somebody, with me. They said they would never forget us. Mum was surprised to realise that my operation had been so unusual to them all. Robert and Caroline Ellis came to see me later on.

Saturday 4th November
I woke feeling a lot better today. I had my drain taken out and then a nice bath. For lunch I had ham and parsley sauce. At 12.45 pm Mr Vernon, the anaesthetist, came especially to see me. I didn't really remember him. Mum was very pleased to see him and took a photo of him and me. He said he was very attached to me. He also said that another patient's operation had had to wait for mine, and the other lady had hers later.

Sunday 5th November
Uncle Eric, Auntie Janette, and Alex and Anna came to see me. I had braised steak for lunch, and I don't need to collect what I do in the bedpan any more. At visiting time it was a nice surprise to see Mum's cousins, Brian and Val and for Mum to catch up with the news about their daughter, Patsy and boyfriend Martin. Ruth brought Hellen and Andrew in later on and we had a nice chat and laugh with them.

Monday 6th November
Dr Fairbrother came round and said he was happy for me to go home today if Dr Sands was OK with it, but he never

came, so I have to have another boring night in hospital. Sister Marie took my stitches out later on, along with an audience of three other nurses as the doctors had used a special different way of sewing me up.

Tuesday 7th November
I had a bath before Dr Fairbrother came round and he said I could definitely go out today, even if Dr Sands didn't come round. Mum packed my case and Dad came in after lunch to take us back. Dr Fairbrother came up to say goodbye; I don't think he wanted me to go really. When we got back home, Uncle Peter called with loads of beautiful flowers. I went to bed early and my bed feels beautiful; it is so soft.

So after a year of invasive and unpleasant tests, Sally, at fifteen years old, had survived a life-threatening experience and was in need of a period of calm to rebuild her strength. We were so grateful and relieved to have her home, and her irrepressible sense of fun very quickly returned.

Wednesday 8th November
I had a wonderful night's sleep and then went into Mum's bed. I kept dozing off throughout the day. Maureen Lucas came to see me about 11 o'clock and stayed while Mum went to the church coffee morning. Peter Holliday came to see me later on and I enjoyed talking to him. I watched the Harvest

Supper entertainment on video and then Marie and Di came to see me with a letter from my class at school.

Thursday 9th November

I had a sleepy sort of a morning and then, around lunchtime, our local doctor came to see me. It was a bit silly as he didn't seem to know anything about me. He took my blood pressure, and said it was fine. I wrote a letter to Ruth Nielson, telling her about everything that had happened. At about 5.30 pm, Juliette and Ruth Holliday came to see me; that was nice. At 8.30 pm I watched 'Some mothers do have 'em'. It was funny (as always!)

Friday 10th November

I had a slightly disturbed night. Cynthia Tipper came to be with me while Mum went off to sort out a new toilet suite. Natalie came round with some flowers and a card later on. I came downstairs for tea and stayed up all evening. I had a few giggling fits today, but not for too long because of my scar!

Saturday 11th November

I came downstairs for breakfast and actually got dressed into my new comfy tracksuit. After lunch I started cutting up old Christmas cards and making them into gift tags for the Christmas bazaar. I made 160 tags so that is 16 bags. I had a sleep in the afternoon.

Wednesday 15th November

Mum took me to Stafford Hospital to see Dr Gibson. He was impressed with my scar, which is ten and a half inches long. He took some blood and then we went to the new Stafford Hospital to see Mr Muir. He changed the wire on my brace and he thinks my teeth are doing fine.

Tuesday 21st November

Mum took me to Lichfield to see Irene Rawe (Sally's flute teacher) and her twin babies, Thomas and Benjamin; they look so different from each other. I had a rest in the afternoon and was full of beans in the evening. I had a bit of a laughing fit at teatime. After tea I did some biology homework and then made some more gift tags (red ones!)

Monday 27th November

I had a homework day and did some of my maths project and also some English. After tea I had a bath and tried to go to bed a bit earlier. Mum and Dad were both out so I did the shouting at the boys!!

Thursday 30th November

I went back to school today and we had French, English, Physics, and Maths. Of course, I enjoyed Maths the most. Mum collected me at lunchtime to prevent me from getting too tired.

Thursday 14th December
I had my first full day back at school today and I took my biology test. After school, I went to the School disco with Marie. I wanted to ask Neil out, then I thought about the last dance, but the last dance was Auld Lang Syne, so I just held hands with him. I really fancy him, so I shall, hopefully, get someone to ask him out for me.

Friday 15th December
Sarah asked Neil out for me but he said no! But he does just want to be good friends. I shall want a mega Christmas kiss from him though!

Wednesday 20th December
We didn't do any work today as it is the last day before the Christmas break. In Chemistry, Mr Nash asked all the girls if anyone could baby-sit for him on New Year's Eve, as he trusted all of us. I thought this was a nice compliment. In the afternoon, Mum took me to see Dr Gibson as he wanted me to have a blood test. This is because since my splenectomy I now have too many platelets, so my blood clots too easily, whereas before I had too few – typical!

Friday 22nd December
Mum and Andrew went out to have their hair cut and do some shopping. I stayed in to look after Robert and do some

ironing. I even managed to get Robert to vacuum and polish his bedroom. Mum and Andrew got back just after 1 o'clock. Mum's hair looks really beautiful. She has had it cut quite short and it looks as if it is bobbed, but it's scrunched dried. It really suits her.

Monday 25th December

We all had lots of presents to open today. We had a yummy Christmas dinner with Grandma and Granddad who are staying with us. I was a bit tired, so I had a rest in the afternoon.

Sunday 31st December

We went to church and I looked after The Kingfishers group on my own. We had a late tea then, after a game of Pictionary, put Robert to bed and then we saw the New Year in. It is now 12.50 am, so I had better get some sleep!

CHAPTER SEVEN

YET ANOTHER GASTROSCOPY

❧

1990

Sally's recovery continued, but the ongoing medical tests were disruptive of her schooling and she was still getting quite tired. She also got very cross at patronising remarks which cast doubt on her abilities and determination, as illustrated in her diary entry of 10th January.

Wednesday 10th January
It was harder to get up this morning, as it was so dark and dingy. At school Chemistry was good as we were dealing with mega poisonous stuff; English was mega boring; and Home Economics was good because I got a lot of work done. After school I had a nice chat with Mum. After Mum went out to W.I., I found a letter from school addressed to Mum and Dad about me. It was about a PATHETIC school medical.

I was really cross because it went on about careers and that I should go to see the rubbish doctor about a career, making sure it would suit my rubbish health. It made me sound as if I couldn't choose my own career. So I was really angry and I am definitely NOT going.

Thursday 11th January
This morning I had no breakfast or anything to drink, which really annoys me. I walked Sam quite early and then Mum took me off to Stafford for yet another gastroscopy. I had the usual very boring wait. Dr Gibson didn't have to inject my veins, so I had a blood test and then went home. I was tired and cross that I had such a pathetic wasted day.

Friday 12th January
I had a lie in this morning. I didn't feel up to school as I was still getting over the effect of the anaesthetic. Judy and Carole came for lunch so that was nice. At 5 o'clock, Di Asplin came to pick up Mum and they went off to give blood. [Val had decided it was time to give back some blood as Sally had received so much.]

Monday 15th January
I was quite pleased with myself today as I felt I had made up for the schoolwork I had missed. In games, it was quite

boring as I was just watching. Next week I am going to do some dance though! After school I went with Mum to her yoga class, which was very relaxing

Sunday 21st January

I got up and did my dog duty and then went off to church to help with the 'Kingfishers'. In the evening I went back to church to the Youth Group. We had a debate on capital punishment and most people were in favour. I strongly disagree. They can't possibly have thought it through if they are in favour.

Saturday 10th February

I got up quite early and went off to Burton with Mum. We bought a pair of super trainers for me and then met up with my cousin, Emma, who I hadn't seen for seven years. It was great seeing her again; she is really lovely and we are going to keep in touch and, hopefully, see her more often.

Wednesday 14th February

I got up early and Mum took me to Stafford to see Dr Gibson. He took some blood and made his usual jokes! I got into school at 9.30 am, just for the end of Chemistry. Mum and Dad went to my parent's evening and they said the teachers were pleased with my work. Pretty good aye!!

Friday 2nd March

I got up very early and at 3.00 am forty of us school kids were on a coach to Manchester on our way to Austria. The plane took off at 7.35am and the flight was OK. When we got to the hotel we unpacked and then had free time until teatime. We walked into the town, which was very quaint.

Wednesday 7th March

We went off skiing at the usual time and our group came down twice this morning. After we got back to the hotel, there was rather a commotion and Natalie was screaming. She had fallen awkwardly and dislocated her knee. I could tell that it was dislocated as the bone was sticking out. The doctor had to whack the bone back into place. Then Natalie was taken to hospital to have her leg put into plaster. Poor old Nat, I feel really sorry for her as she is in a lot of pain.

Thursday 8th March

This is our last day of skiing. We went down the run twice this morning and then, after lunch, we went down three times more; the second time I went really, really fast. We had the marks for our presentations later on. I got level 5, which is the lowest, but I don't care!!

Friday 9th March

We had to get up early this morning to have breakfast, and then off to the airport to fly home. The flight took two hours and the landing was bumpy because of strong winds. After two hours on the coach we arrived back in Lichfield, and Mum was waiting for me. When I got back home, Mum had decorated my bedroom; the wallpaper on the cupboard had been changed to match my quilt and it's beautiful. Mum had also put up some shelves, which are great. It's really super to be home.

Sunday 11th March
I got up and walked Sam, then we all went to church, but it wasn't Peter, so we had quite a dozy vicar. After church I made some soup and then we spent time in the garden, as it was such a nice day. I had some crackers and cheese for supper, and discovered that I like blue cheese!

Sunday 18th March
It was a beautiful day and we went to church. Afterwards a very pregnant Judy and family came round for lunch and stayed all afternoon; it was really pleasant. In the evening I went with the youth group to Stafford Superbowl for ten-pin bowling. It was great fun even though I wasn't very good!

Tuesday 20th March
Douglas rang first thing this morning to say that Judy had

given birth to a baby girl at 2.34 am this morning weighing 7lb 8oz, and everything is fine. School wasn't very exciting but Marianne was on cloud nine because Simon had asked her out and she said yes! I walked the dogs after tea and then had a nice bubbly bath.

Friday 23rd March

In Chemistry I had to do a spoken test and I was dead nervous but I managed (I don't know how!) but I got a special! After school, Grandma and Granddad were over with the Friday Club. After they had gone home, I took Felicity back to Judy's house and stayed for ages so I could have a good cuddle with the baby, who still hasn't got a name! Mum and Dad went out in the evening and I made a Mother's Day cake.

Monday 26th March

Not a very exciting day at school. After school, I took my maths project round to Judy's so I could ask some questions. Judy was feeding the baby at the time. (She still hasn't officially got a name yet!) Later on Mum and I went to our yoga class and I fell asleep during the deep relax.

Tuesday 27th March

At school today I had an interview with Ms Clark. She was just asking me how my subjects are going. After school, I did some homework and then walked the dogs with Dad. Later on, I put 'ELIZABETH' on the embroidery I am doing even though Judy and Douglas haven't officially announced the baby's name, because Judy is pretty sure that's what it's going to be!

Thursday 29th March

I handed my maths projects in today and it was a great feeling that I had got it out of the way! In Physics I sat next to Neil, which is great fun because he is such a laugh. After school I went to the optician's. He did an ace test by putting some dye in my eyes. It was great fun. It has been officially announced that Judy's baby is called Elizabeth Mary. I finished the sampler, framed it, and took it round to Judy. She was thrilled to bits.

Wednesday 11th April

I had a lie in! I always get up when I hear the postman, but when I came down it was the milkman! So I went back to bed again.

Thursday 12th April

I suggested to Mum that we go to Birmingham today, but as she was still in bed, she turned her nose up at the thought, but when she got up, she changed her mind. So Mum and I took Sarah Grew and we had a great time. Sarah bought herself a pink dress, some material and a purse for her Mum's birthday. I bought a rather jazzy swimming costume.

Saturday 14th April

I went off to Lichfield with Dad and Robert and bought a £5 record token for Andrew's birthday, and various other birthday cards. At 8.00 pm, Carole, Jason, Peter, Ruth, Douglas, Judy, and Elizabeth came round for a meal and a game of cards. Peter had to go off to the cathedral to do a service and came back at about 11.30pm. Elizabeth woke up at midnight. She was passed around in between her feeds and then, at about 1 am she smiled at Judy. We are all sure it was a real smile.

Friday 20th April

I went to Sue's for the morning, and after lunch, Maureen collected me to have a fitting for my bridesmaid dress. It is very expensive but it is beautiful. When I got home I was tired but at 5.30 pm we went to the swimming baths to take part in a sponsored swim for St James' School. I did 42 widths in 15 minutes and really enjoyed myself.

Tuesday 24th April

Mum opened her birthday presents in bed this morning. She

had a carving knife from Andrew, a book and a sexy swimming costume from Dad, and a small kitchen knife from me. I had a horrible day at school and had a good cry on Mum later. I hope I didn't spoil her birthday. After tea I walked the dogs with Dad and then babysat Elizabeth for Judy. I fed her and changed her nappy. She was very good and I thought I coped really well.

Wednesday 25th April

I didn't enjoy school at all today. When I got home, Mum had had her interview at Tamworth College and she's got a job. I am really pleased for her. I didn't do much in the evening because I was depressed from a yucky day, but Dad made me laugh with his funny little ways!!

Sunday 3rd June

After the church service this morning, Judy and Douglas asked Dad if he would be a godfather for Elizabeth, and, of course, he said yes. After lunch, Peter came down to tell me that Liz's wedding was cancelled, so I was a bit upset, but after a while I got over it. I spent most of the rest of the day reading and revising.

Monday 11th June

School was boring today, as usual. After school I went to the shop to buy a card for Cathy, because yesterday her dad, John Furniss, was killed in an accident on his bike. In the evening I went to my yoga class, but Mum didn't come as she had a boring school governor's meeting. I really enjoyed it.

Wednesday 15th August
Mum and Dad's 20th Wedding Anniversary
I got up early and gave Mum and Dad a present and anniversary card, and then had a shower to wake me up. Just before 8.00 am Mum and I popped off to Stafford District Hospital to have yet another gastroscopy. I had a local anaesthetic but it had an hypnotic drug in it, so that I wouldn't remember the gastroscopy, and I didn't remember; I was fine. I slept for about an hour and then saw Dr Gibson. We then went home and both went to bed for a little sleep. In the evening, we listened to Mum and Dad's wedding tape. On the Jimmy Young's radio 2 show in the morning, he played a record for Mum and Dad; it was super. Dad had written in two weeks earlier.

Saturday 15th September
When I got up, Mum told me that Sam had pinched my apple and blackcurrant pie last night. Obviously I was cross, but I went straight down stairs and made another one! I took all my eleven exhibits up to the village hall produce show for 10.30 am. At 2.00 pm I went back to see if I had won

anything. I came first with my fruit pie, blackcurrant jam, lemon curd, vase of flowers, vegetable animal, jam tarts, cheese scones, and butterfly cakes. I came second with my Victoria sponge, but I didn't come anywhere with my savoury flan, and fruitcake.

Monday 8th October
Work Experience.
Dad took me to the Good Hope Hospital and we arrived at the pharmacy at 8.00 am. First, I delivered some controlled drugs to the wards, including ITU; it was very busy there. I actually made up quite a lot of prescriptions, and I had to keep looking for the drugs; it was great fun. I really enjoyed my days work, but I was really, really tired afterwards.

Tuesday 9th October
I got to the hospital a bit earlier, and helped pack some drugs and things that the theatre needed. One of the things I packed was a liquid, and the pharmacist said 'don't drop that otherwise we will all fall asleep'. I made up two prescriptions that were quite large, and I didn't have any supervision at all. In the afternoon, I went over to the school of nursing and watched a video about a drug called TPA, which is used when a patient has a heart attack, to unblock the clogged up artery. The drug costs £600 a dose!! I came home on the train, had tea and then walked the dogs.

Thursday 11ᵗʰ October
I had a really ace day today. I made up a box of drugs for the theatre and then I went with Cynthia to make some pessaries. We made them in the aseptic room where it is completely sterile. We had to put on a blue sterile gown, gloves, shoe coverings, hat, and mask. It was ace fun! I made up loads of prescriptions as they were quite short staffed.

Saturday 13ᵗʰ October
I had a really long lie in. but I still wasn't awake when I got up! The electricians were here all day, and my room is in a MEGA MESS.

Monday 15ᵗʰ October
School was really boring in comparison to work experience. After school, the electrician was still here working in my bedroom, so I had to do my homework downstairs.

Thursday 18ᵗʰ October
Mum collected me from school at 10.30 am and we went to Stafford Hospital to see Dr Gibson. We had to wait for nearly two hours. I had a chat to him about being interested in pharmacy, and he is going to write to the Royal Pharmaceutical Society explaining my condition. I had a blood test, and then we had some Kentucky fried chicken. It was yummy. We were too late to go back to school, so I did some work at home.

Friday 19ᵗʰ October
School was OK today, and I handed in two science assessments. In drama we had to clean out the back room, so only did a bit of acting. In the evening, I babysat for Judy. Sarah has got chickenpox, and looks really poorly. Elizabeth woke up and made a racket for a while, and was a bit of a rogue.

Monday 12ᵗʰ November
School was fine today. Maths was good and I didn't do any work in English as I was busy talking. After tea, Mum collected Juliette Holliday from Judy's and took us both to the Vicarage, and I am stopping the night, as Ruth has a bad back and has to stay in bed.

Wednesday 14ᵗʰ November
I woke up a little earlier at Ruth's this morning. I fed the dogs and then fed Ruth!! Well, took her some toast up. Dad collected me and took me to school. In the evening, Mum gave me a relaxing massage as I wasn't in a very good mood.

Friday 16ᵗʰ November
After school, Ruth came round with a present for looking after her. It was a purple and grey jumper with two penguins on the front; it's beautiful. I suggested that we all go for a walk with the dogs, so we did. It was really windy and we were all really daft!!

Tuesday 20th November

I went to school today despite having an aching back. It was hard going and I didn't do PE. There was an election today, as Mr Heseltine wants to become the Prime Minister. The votes were 204 for Mrs Thatcher and 152 for Mr Heseltine. A second vote is needed, so Mrs Thatcher might not be Prime minister for much longer; but I hope she is.

Thursday 22nd November
Mrs Thatcher's Resignation

I went to school But it was really foggy and generally a yucky day. During English we heard that Mrs Thatcher has resigned from being Prime Minister. Personally, I wish she hadn't. After school I was exhausted and had a rest before doing some more of my Maths project.

Tuesday 27th November
New Prime Minister

Firstly, we had assembly; it was OK. We then had Geography and we didn't do much. In the afternoon we had French, and we were in the language lab. I got a fit of the giggles for no apparent reason! At 6.30pm the results of the election were announced between John Major, Douglas Hurd, and Michael Heseltine. John Major won, but he needed another two votes to win outright, but, because the other two pulled out, he is now the new Prime Minister.

Friday 30ᵗʰ November

School went with a bang!(Only a figure of speech!) Mr Caldwell was particularly complimentary today, calling me 'Mature'! After school, I made some ginger beer with an attentive audience (Granddad). After tea I walked the dogs with Granddad. He told me some stories about the war that were really, really funny.

Saturday 8ᵗʰ December
Snow!

We woke up to a blizzard this morning. At 11.30 am, the electricity went off. By this time the snow was really deep and, after lunch, we went outside and played in the snow with the dogs. Later on, Judy and Douglas and the children came round for tea and we spent a candlelit evening together. We had good fun.

Sunday 16ᵗʰ December
We all went to church and I thought it was very boring. The Bishop of Lichfield was there to present the Bishop Certificate people with their certificates. Dad got a merit on his. (What a boff!!) After lunch, Robert went to a Christmas party at church. They had to dress up and so he went as Santa Claus! Mum and dad had a secret wrapping up session in their bedroom. I am getting more and more nervous about my

exams this week. We watched the comedy awards in the evening and had a good laugh.

Monday 24th December
Mum and Dad got up early and went shopping, and then Dad went to get Grandma and Granddad. Andrew and Robert walked the dogs and Sam bit Robert on the leg. We took him straight to the hospital and he had to have a few stitches. He was very brave. I went with Mum and Dad to midnight mass and it was a lovely service. I am now very tired and I'm going to put my light out before Santa comes!

Tuesday 25th December
I woke up at 7.15 am and we all did our usual transportation into Mum and Dad's room to open our presents. Jonathan Dudley and Paula called in the afternoon and stayed for a while for a lovely chat. I bathed Robert in the evening, but he had to keep his leg up so that he didn't get his plaster wet. I am now very tired and so is everyone else! I think everyone will be having a lie in tomorrow.

Monday 31st December
I was up amazingly early and Dad went off to work. The rest of us went off to Sutton Coldfield for a very good shop. In the evening, Mum and Dad went to Judy's mum and dad's for a new year's party. I went off to a party and stayed the night at Tina's.

CHAPTER EIGHT

THE SHOW WENT BRILLIANTLY

❧

1991

Tuesday 15th January
We performed an extract of our 'Grease' show in assembly in front of the 5th and 6th form. It went well. Quite a lot of people are worried at school about war in Iraq, which may start tomorrow. In the evening mum and I finished making the capes for the 'Grease' production.

Wednesday 16th January
I stayed after school for a 'Grease' rehearsal, but it wasn't very successful. I was in somewhat of a depressed mood all evening, because I don't feel very well and things are getting too much for me.

Thursday 17th January
War broke out during the night in Iraq, and at the moment

the battle is only from the air, and quite a lot of targets have been hit by US troops. News updates are going on all the time (it's scary). Mum and Dad went to a meeting at school for parents of prospective 6th form students. I made Robert's birthday cake for tomorrow.

Friday 18th January
Robert's birthday
The war is still going on and loads of reports from Baghdad keep coming in. After school, I helped with Robert's football party at the Village Hall. Mum gave blood today as lots of people are needed to give because of the Gulf crisis.

Monday 21st January
The war is continuing in Iraq and now some of our men have been taken hostage. We had a full 'Grease' rehearsal at lunchtime. After school, I didn't feel very well and actually fell asleep.

Wednesday 23rd January
We had the 'Grease' dress rehearsal today and it went really well. During English we had a stupid cop talking about drink driving. I told him that it was very boring!

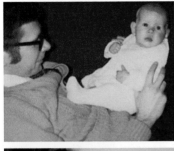
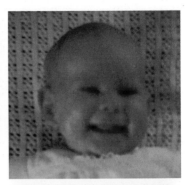
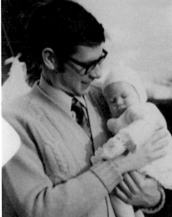
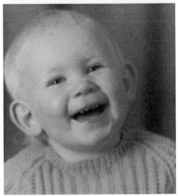

1974-75 - one happy baby

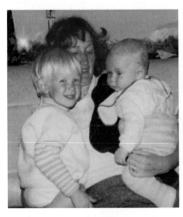
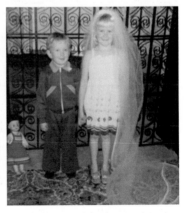

Aged two, with baby brother Andrew   Playing weddings, aged five

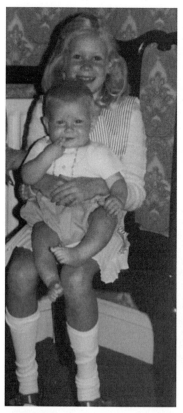

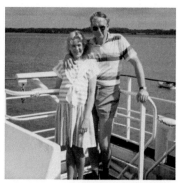

Age 11, on a ferry with Dad

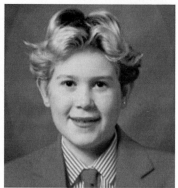

Age seven - Robert's second mum

Age 12 in her first year at
the Friary School

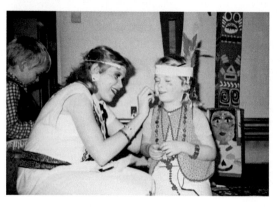

Age 12, dressing
Sarah up for
Robert's fifth
birthday party

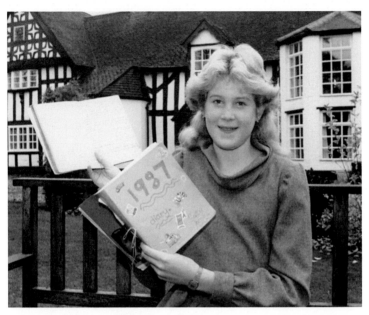

Sally's diary writing and Margaret Seddon's diary of 1864 made the local newspaper when she was 13 (1987)

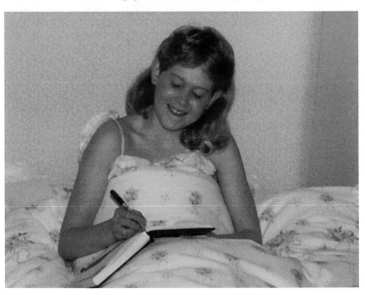

Writing her diary at bedtime (1988)

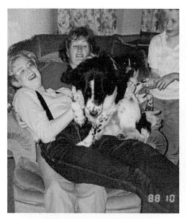

Sam and Lucky gatecrash the
armchair (1988)

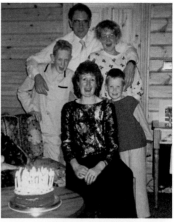

Mum's 40th birthday

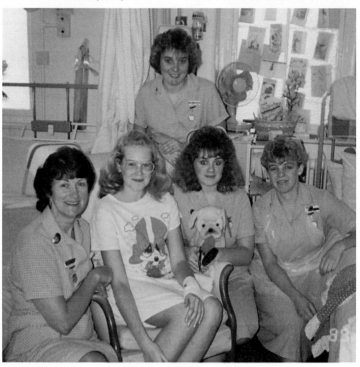

October 1989 - at Mansfield Hospital, recovering from her emergency
splenectomy

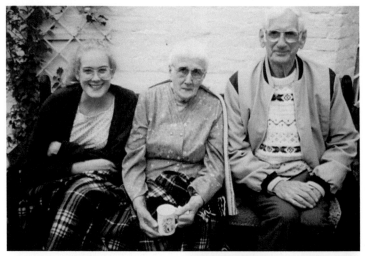

Resting with Grandma and Granddad
in the garden, August 1994

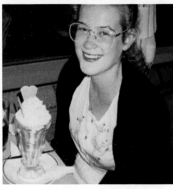

A few weeks pre-transplant, July 1994

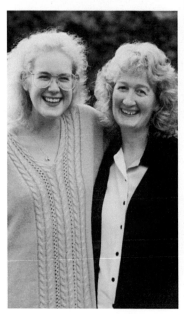

Sept 1994 - two weeks
post liver transplant

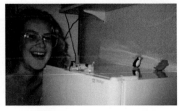

20th birthday, October 1994.
Humping dog sitting on my new
fridge. Penguin walks away in disgust!
(Three weeks post transplant)

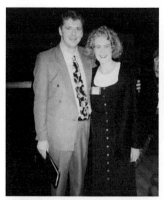

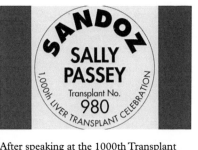

After speaking at the 1000th Transplant
Celebrations at Birmingham University,
March 1995, with Anthony Hooker,
Transplant Co-ordinator.

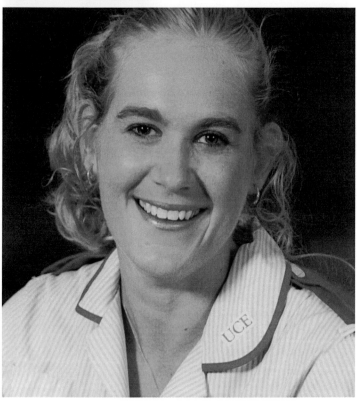

On a Project 2000 nursing course at the University of Central England,
Birmingham, 1995-98

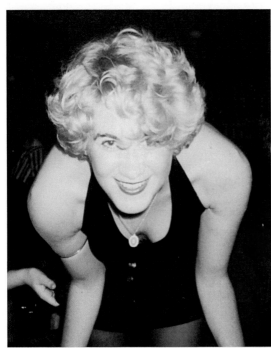

'I have so much
energy with a
new liver!'

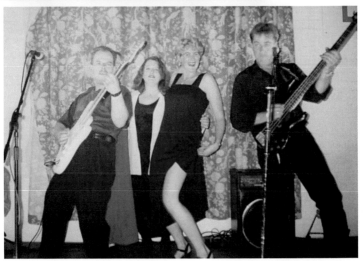

Helping out with the band at a dance at Longdon Village Hall, 1996

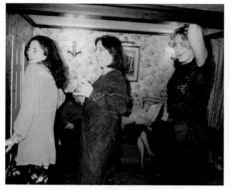

Wild dancing at midnight with Judy and
Carole, New Year's Eve 1996

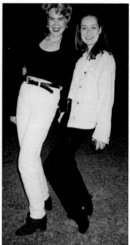

Looking chic with Lindsey

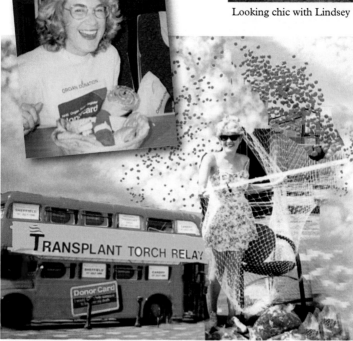

Promoting the donor card, in Centenary Square Birmingham, 1996 (above)
and on the train to London, and back to Birmingham in Transplant week 1997

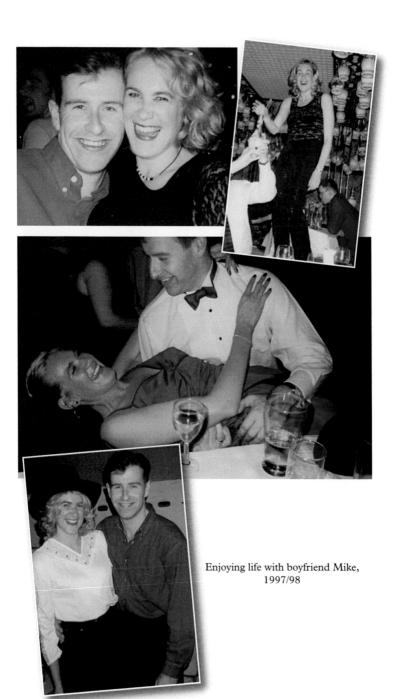

Enjoying life with boyfriend Mike,
1997/98

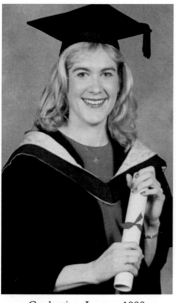

Graduation, January 1999

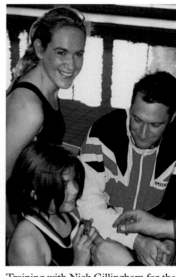

Training with Nick Gillingham for the
British Transplant Games in
Birmingham, June 1999

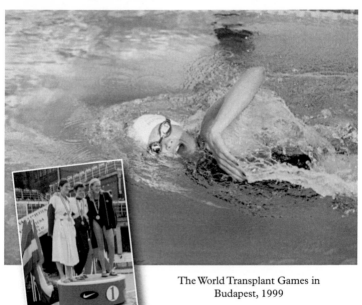

The World Transplant Games in
Budapest, 1999

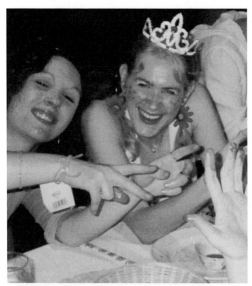

Little Miss Sunshine's hen party, 2000

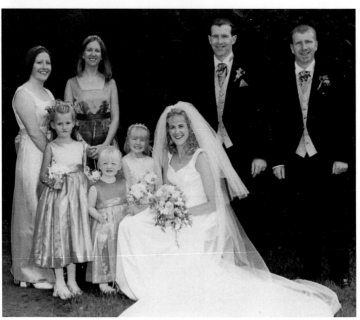

Sally and Mike's Rainbow Wedding, 16th September 2000

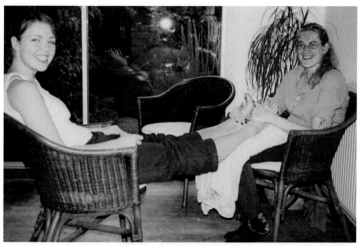

Practising reflexology on Rachel

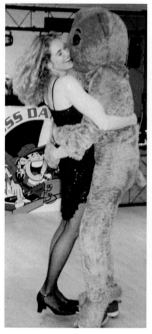

Bearhug from Rob on his
21st birthday in 2003

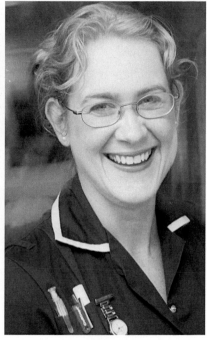

Sister Sally Painting

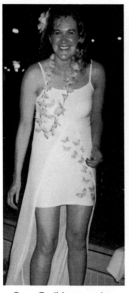

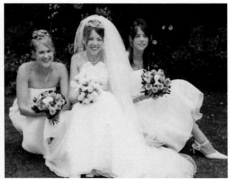

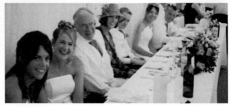

On a Caribbean cruise,
2004

Bridesmaid at Andrew and Rachel's wedding,
May 2004

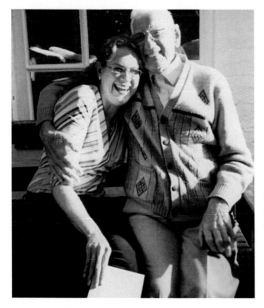

A big hug from
Granddad after
showing him the baby
scan, September 2004

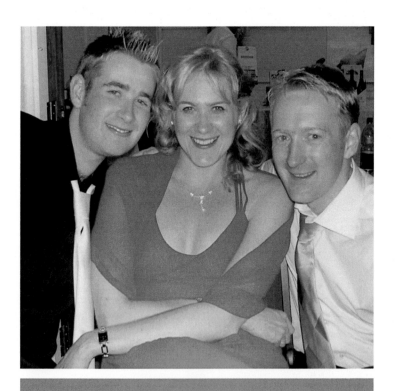

Dear...**Grandad**..

You are invited to a Dinner Dance to celebrate

**Sally's 30th Birthday and the
10 year Anniversary of her Liver Transplant.**

On 9th October 2004
7pm
at Longdon Village Hall, Brook End, Longdon, nr Lichfield

Dress: Black tie.
(Boys you can get away with jacket and tie. Girls wear anything sparkly and glam!!)
Bring your own drink

The best party ever - 7th October 2004

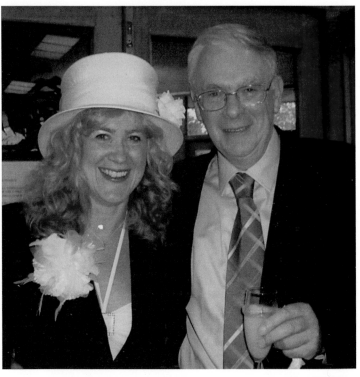

At Hellen Holliday's wedding in October 2004, one of the
last pictures taken of Sally

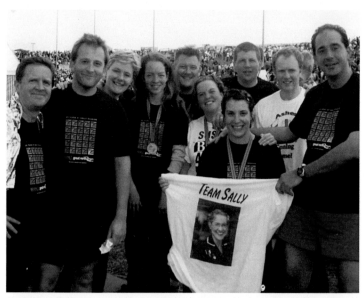

Hospital staff do the Great North Run in Sally's memory, September 2005

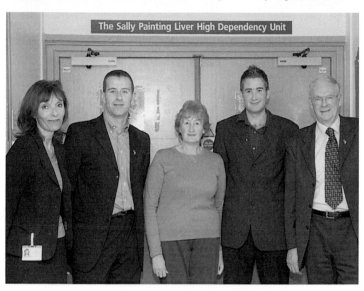

Maggie Bayley, assistant director of nursing, and members of the family at the naming of the Sally Painting Liver High Dependency Unit

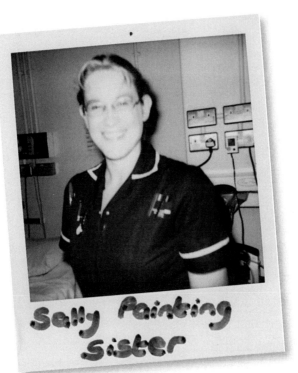

Sally Painting
Sister

Thursday 24th January
GREASE
I excused myself from the last two lessons so I could help get the lecture theatre ready for tonight. Everything went really well and we were all really tired afterwards. I had better get to sleep now or I will be knackered for tomorrow.

Friday 25th January
I couldn't concentrate at school today. Loads of people were commenting about last night's performance. It was brill! So what if Colin did a load of ad libs, it was still very funny.

Saturday 26th January
Last night of Grease
Mum collected Emma from the station and we all had a pub lunch. In the evening the show went BRILLIANTLY and we all had a party afterwards. I got my programme signed by everyone, including Richard, the yummy drummer, and Andy Barber! I had a kiss from Andy and we all had an ace time.

Wednesday 6th February
I spoke to Mr Firth today about pharmacy as a career and he was really helpful. In the evening I went to a careers convention at school. It was really good and I gathered a lot of information.

Friday 8th February
School was cancelled today because of heavy snow. I took the
sledge out and gave Sarah a ride. After lunch, all our family,
plus the dogs, went sledging up the field. I took the dogs down
on the sledge. It was really funny!

On Friday 15th February, Sally went with the church young people's group to a weekend in Wales.

Saturday 16th February
We had a busy day mountain climbing and I felt quite faint
in the evening. We all went down to the village and on the
way back our lads were set upon by some local youths. A
policeman came and we all had to give statements. Very
upsetting.

The incident involved returning to Wales for a court hearing. The youths were troublemakers known to the police.

Wednesday 27th February
Dad took me to the hospital today for a gastroscopy. It was
fine. Mum collected me later as I can now sign myself in! I
went to sleep in the afternoon.

Tuesday 19th March
I had a day off school today as I fell down the stairs and hurt my back. Mum sent for the doctor, but he didn't think it was serious. He told me to rest on my back, which is very boring.

Thursday 21st March
Mum took me to Stafford Hospital and I had an x-ray and saw Dr Gibson. He said there was nothing wrong apart from bruising. Dad has written a letter to Michael Heseltine about the poll tax. It's brill!!

I can't remember what I wrote, but the gist of it was that I didn't think it was a good idea.

Friday 29th March
I went up to church and there was a TV crew filming. They interviewed me about my views on advertising the church. On the early evening news they didn't show the interview, but the camera panned right in on me! It is ace. I kept watching the video recording and I couldn't stop laughing about it!

Saturday 27th April
We spent all day in the garden working on the trees. If I wasn't shredding I was chopping. It was a beautiful day. We had chicken and chips for tea and ate them in the garden. I then had a well-earned bath.

Saturday 4th May

We went to London on a coach, and after we had checked in at our hotel, we went to Harrods and then had a walk through the park. At 7.45 pm we watched Aspects of Love at the Prince of Wales theatre. It was excellent and I really enjoyed it.

Monday 1st July

I had a lie in this morning, which was really nice. I then watched a bit of Wimbledon and went to work at Sue's in the afternoon. The new law for having to wear seat belts in the back of cars came into force today. In the evening I went to choir practice.

Tuesday 2nd July

After walking the dogs, Judy dropped Elizabeth off at our house. She is so cute and can now say quite a few words. I sunbathed while watching the tennis later on. Edberg beat McEnroe, which I was pleased about because he is bosting.

Thursday 4th July

I went to see Dr Gibson today and he said that I might have to see a gynaecologist because I haven't started yet. It was a really hot day. I wrote three letters and also did some mounting of flowers. In the evening I babysat for the Grews' children. They were all very good.

Thursday 11th July
It was the school sports day today. I served ice-cream and cold drinks with Mum, and we did a great trade as it was a beautiful day. At 9.15 pm I babysat for the Grews' children again. Sarah stayed up quite late for a chat. She is so sweet and always thinks of me as a sister, which makes me feel quite honoured.

Saturday 13th July
Dad and I went into Lichfield and had a good look around Texas. It poured with rain in the afternoon, so I did some work on my new jacket. At around 7 pm, Uncle Peter and Auntie Joan and family came over and we all went to the Lichfield Festival fireworks. They were fantastically, beautifully, amazingly, trendy!

Tuesday 16th July
We looked after Elizabeth this morning and when we went shopping, she fell asleep in the trolley! I went to work at Sue's in the afternoon, and was quite busy serving in the shop. I babysat for Carole in the evening.

Thursday 15th August
Mum and Dad's 21st wedding anniversary
I spent the day preparing the meal for tonight. I did tomato soup, cod with spicy sauce, honeyed pork and hazelnut galette.

I did it all without Mum knowing. Dad bought Mum an amethyst pendant with matching earrings, and Mum bought Dad cufflinks with his initials engraved on them. Both were from the same shop, so they had the same boxes, which was really funny!

Saturday 17th August
Mum took me to Burton and I spent the day with Emma, and then we went back to her house in Nottingham. In the evening we watched the film 'Ghost', and I cried because it was so sad. I am staying for a couple of days.

Thursday 22nd August
GCSE RESULTS
I got 'B's in English, Science, and Home Economics; a 'C' in Geography; and 'D's in Maths and French. I was very disappointed. At 1.00 pm I was at Stafford Hospital for a gastroscopy. The nurses on the ward were really mardy today. We had a Chinese takeaway for tea, which was really YUM.

After the disappointment of her GCSE results, we all went off for a week's holiday in Scotland. Sally was still keen to carry on doing 'A' levels and decided to study chemistry, English, maths, and biology.

Sunday September 1st

I went to church but had a depressing day thinking about tomorrow and the court case [the Welsh thugs]. *Nathalie came round later and we had a good chat about exam results. I watched a good film in the evening, but it had a silly ending.*

Monday September 2nd

I had to get up early and Mum and Dad took me to the court at Caernarfon. The rest of our youth group were there as we were witnesses. We weren't needed as the youths pleaded guilty at the last minute. It was an exhausting day and when we got home I went to see Judy for a chat.

Tuesday September 3rd

Back to school. I'm a 6th former and it's great having our own base. I have seven free lessons a week. This afternoon I had chemistry with Mrs Broad.

Wednesday September 4th

I had biology with Mrs Beer. She is really nice. In the evening I watched the recorded 'Hospital Watch'.

Over the next three weeks Sally went to see an endocrinologist with the inevitable blood test, had a visit from our own doctor with a suspected kidney infection, and saw her consultant, Dr Gibson, for a thorough examination and ultrasound scan.

Wednesday 25th September

I stayed in bed again all morning and then felt a bit better. Dad has had a word with the doctor and he wants me to see a gynaecologist, so I am going into hospital tomorrow.

Thursday 26th September

I got up and had a bath and then Mum took me to Stafford Hospital. I didn't see a doctor all day, but what has kept me going is a lovely hunky lad I can see through my window! I have to stay the night. BORING!! Judy came in to see me.

Friday 27th September

I had a boring day in hospital and a very degrading experience that a gynaecologist carried out on me, and it hurt! Dad and Andrew came in to see me. I am really pissed off, if you will excuse the expression.

Sunday 29th September

I had a boring morning but, after lunch, Mr Daniels, the gynaecologist, came to see me and said I could go home. I immediately phoned Mum, but she had already left to visit me. I packed my bags and, when Mum came, we had to wait for my pills, and then we went home. It's lovely to be back home.

Tuesday 1st October
After a lie in and a shower, I went into school at break-time.

I had a lot of copying up to do but I felt a lot better. After school, Dad came home as he has had a wisdom tooth out. Poor old Dad!

Thursday 3rd October
I have done so much writing today; I'm surprised my hand hasn't dropped off. I had a parcel through the post; it's a birthday present!!

Saturday 5th October
I had a shower and then Alex and Anna came to stay for the weekend. At 10.00 am I started my new Saturday job at Boots the chemists. I just had training today. My uniform is really smart.

Monday 7th October
My 17th Birthday
I had loads of presents including a watch. School was OK. I had a whole string of visitors after school bringing me presents and cards. We had a power cut for over two hours, which was very exciting. My birthday cake is an L-plate.

Thursday 10th October
I had to go and see Dr Gibson today and we had to wait for ages. I got back to school for 15 minutes of biology and a double free in the afternoon. I was at Boots after school, working on the till, and later on I babysat for the Grews.

Sunday 20th October
I served at church today and it was really cold. When we got back, I made some soup for lunch. After lunch, Dad took me out for a driving lesson! It's harder than you think. I haven't quite mastered the clutch and accelerator movement yet. I listened to the charts when I got back, and Bryan Adams is still number one for the 16th week. I have been knitting a jumper for a child in India.

Tuesday 22nd October
Work shadowing a dietician at Stafford Hospital
I had to get up early to catch a bus to Stafford. I had a great day visiting the wards and seeing patients, including a tiny baby being fed nasalgastrically. When I got home I felt whacked, so I watched TV all evening.

Saturday 26th October
I had an early morning wake up from Felicity as I had stayed the night at the Grews. I was at work at Boots by 10.00 am (I sold my first pack of condoms and I didn't go bright red!)

Saturday 2nd November
I was on the early shift at Boots and it got busy quite quickly. At lunchtime, I had a look at some ball gowns but have come to the conclusion that buying some material would be better.

Monday 11th November

I struggled through the morning trying not to think about the maths exam this afternoon. It wasn't too bad and at least I managed to finish the paper. Mum collected me after school and I had a nap before doing some homework. In the evening, Mum started sewing my ball gown. It's ACE!

Monday 18th November

I didn't enjoy school today, as I got a rubbish mark for my biology essay. After school, I went to the doctors to see about my non-bendable thumb. Dr Abbott is referring me to someone at Stafford. Terry Waite has been freed after five years in captivity in Beirut.

Thursday 21st November

School was OK. Mr Tyler went over some points in biology and made it easier to understand. I had a driving lesson after school and I ventured into the town. It was great and I did loads of roundabouts as well. When I got home, Mum had finished my dress. It's BRILLIANT.

Wednesday 11th December

School was a laugh today and went amazingly fast. In the evening I went to Ruskin's restaurant for the Boots Christmas meal. It was really good fun, and I sat by Mr John, the manager. We had a really good laugh.

Saturday 14th December

I was on the early shift at Boots and I worked on the counter all the time. Dad collected me afterwards and told me that Sam had bitten another dog, so it was a bit fraught at home. I made some mince pies with Mum. James came down to play with Andrew on the computer. Andrew has got a bad groin, but it is better than it was yesterday.

Sunday 15th December

We arrived late at church and Jonathan and Paula were there. [They had recently left Longdon and moved to Leamington]. *They came back to our house for lunch, and we had a lovely time. They have invited us to visit them in the New Year. I wrapped up all my Christmas presents later on.*

Tuesday 24th December

I had to get up early as I worked all day at Boots. It went quite fast and I really enjoyed myself. I dropped off to sleep after tea and, later on, I went with Mum and Dad to Midnight Mass. It was lovely.

Tuesday 31ˢᵗ December

I still felt a bit groggy today. I worked at Boots from 10.00am till 4.00pm, which did me in somewhat, but I coped. There was a dishy pharmacist on today called Bob! It was just our family celebrating New Year. We had a lovely time playing games and being silly.

CHAPTER NINE

CAN I VIDEO MY GASTROSCOPY PLEASE?

1992

Wednesday 1ˢᵗ January

We went to Coventry today to take Andy and his mates to a football match. We wandered around Coventry looking at the shops and the cathedral. When we got back home, we went round to the Grews and ended up inviting them round for tea. Elizabeth is so cute and she can count now!

Friday 3ʳᵈ January

I had a lie in and then woke myself up with a shower. I did some more work on my English essay, which is now nearly complete. At 12.00 I went to work at Boots and spent most of the time on the chemist counter. Dad collected me afterwards and when I got home, Mum and I cooked a Chinese meal in my new wok. It was great fun and we all really enjoyed it. Later on we had a game of word square and Dad and I won as we played in pairs.

Saturday 4th January

Dad got me up to take me to Boots at Lichfield; otherwise I could have slept all day! I worked from 10.00 till 4.00 and someone gave me a £20 note that we wouldn't accept as we thought it was forged. After work, Mum and Dad picked me up and we went to Chris and Peter Cooke's house for tea. We had a good time and played some good games.

Tuesday 7th January

I spent most of the morning reading 'Jude' and then, after lunch, Mum took me for a driving lesson. I drove all the way to Marchington and back, even down the big 12% hill. We had a yummy Chinese meal for tea and then, after Robert had gone to bed, Mum and I went round to Judy's, which was nice.

Saturday 11th January

We all went to Jonathan and Paula's house in Leamington Spa. We had coffee and then walked into town. Andrew bought a new coat and I bought an illuminated globe for Robert's birthday next week. After lunch we went for a walk in the park and saw loads of deer. We got back home at 8 pm and I didn't feel too good.

Sunday 12th January

I still felt groggy this morning so I stayed in bed while Mum and Dad went to church. I managed a little soup at lunchtime but didn't feel up to doing much. Later on I watched a football match on television with Andy and Robert!! Wow! It was quite a good match.

Wednesday 15th January
Mr Martin said that the maths results had come so we all charged off to get them. I got a 'C' and was thrilled. I couldn't wait to tell Mum and Dad so I phoned them. After school Mum had put a big sign up congratulating me.

Saturday 18th January
I worked from 10.00 till 4.00 at Boots while Mum and Dad took Robert and his friend to watch Aston Villa. Robert had a goalie shirt for his birthday. Villa lost. Later on I went to Heather's party and we had a great laugh.

Wednesday 29th January
Mum picked me up from school and I drove to Stafford Hospital to see the gynaecologist. It was OK; at least he didn't go poking me around! I have got to see him again in a year's time. I did a bit of homework after tea, but I was really tired.

Tuesday 4th February
I had to get up really early and be on a coach at school for

7.00 am! All the A level English students went to London to a conference. We attended three lectures and, for the rest of the time, dossed around London. We chatted up policemen guarding the gates of Downing Street, visited Westminster Abbey, and walked by the Houses of Parliament. We got back at about 7.15 pm after having a great laugh on the coach.

Thursday 6th February
School was really busy today and we had a great laugh with Mr Forster. I stayed after school for a West Side Story rehearsal. In the evening I watched a TV programme about the Queen called Elizabeth R. It was really good. She has been on the throne for 40 years now.

Wednesday 12th February
I was sick of going into the girls' toilets today and finding smokers in there, so I complained about it and, hopefully, they will be chucked out. We had a lady come to talk to us about higher education and she was very interesting. After tea, Dad and I walked the dogs and then Mum helped me with my homework.

Thursday 13th February
In Chemistry, I had to give a talk with Heather but it wasn't too bad. Mum picked me up and we went to see Dr Gibson. I drove! I asked him if they could video my next gastroscopy and he said that, hopefully, they could.

Friday 14th February
I didn't get any Valentine's cards! Never mind! I had my third driving lesson and when I got back into school I helped Mrs Beer with the second years. We had a right laugh in Biology because I painted Marcus's nails with Tippex when he wasn't looking.

Monday 17th February
When I got home from school, there was no one in as they had all gone to the dentist. I got a bit upset later on, as Chemistry is getting me down. I didn't feel like any tea, so I went with Mum to her yoga class and really enjoyed it. Afterwards we watched the ice-skating on television and it was beautiful.

Wednesday 19th February
I never seem to feel really good in the mornings and I didn't feel brilliant in Biology. After Biology we had English, which was so boring I nearly fell asleep. I practised some dance steps in the afternoon for the West Side Story production and a fifth year boy called Chris Hammersly helped me.

Thursday 27th February
I drove Mum, Andy, and Robert to Burton for a spot of shopping. It was quite distracting with the boys being noisy in the back. I bought a pair of black jeans for only £6.99!

I was knackered when I got home so I had a snooze. After tea, we watched a really good episode of 'Casualty' about a plane crash.

Monday 2nd March
Back to school. I had a chemistry practical test, which was rather boring, as we couldn't use the really reactive chemicals. Mrs Craig liked my skirt that Mum has made for West Side Story. After school I watched a West Side Story video, and then phoned Granddad for a chat. He is so funny.

Wednesday 4th March
We had a biology practical first thing and the rats have arrived, so we may be starting on them next week. In General Studies, Mr Adams asked who believed in sex before marriage. Everyone put their hands up except Tina and me so there will be a discussion on that next week! I have been very good so far with my Lenten discipline of not eating between meals. (Except fruit!)

Thursday 5th March
I was in a good mood at school today, until I was filled with horror when Mr Tyler told us we would be dissecting rats tomorrow. I was a bit cross when he said we shouldn't wear gloves. Anyway, after lunch, our West Side Story mob went to perform in a dance festival. It was good fun and we continued our rehearsals back at school.

Friday 6th March

I had a driving lesson with John Hicks today and he was very reassuring. In the last lesson at school we started the dissection of the rats. Mine is a female and I had to massage its limbs in order to pin it to the board! It wasn't half as bad as I thought it would be.

Tuesday 10th March

Today is our dress rehearsal and it took us ages to get all our make-up done. We had an interval at lunchtime when we paraded around school in our costumes. It was a great laugh. After school I dropped off to sleep, but we have had an excellent day.

Wednesday 11th March

I only had double biology at school and did homework for the rest of the morning. In the afternoon I helped tidy up the back room, ready for tonight's performance. Auntie Barbara and Clare came to watch, and the performance went really well.

Friday 13th March

I had an excellent driving lesson, and joined the main dual carriageway on a slip road. It was ace! In Biology we pulled the guts out of our rats. It was disgusting! After school, I had a little doze before changing for the evening show. Labour MP, Sylvia Heal was in the audience and spoke to us after the show.

Saturday 14th March

I worked all day at Boots and then went into school for the final performance. We had a party at Lisa's afterwards, and I am well knackered now. It is 1.15 am!

Sunday 22nd March

I had a very welcome lie in this morning, and then I did some homework, before going to Peter and Joan's for Granddad's 75th birthday party. Dad and I popped off to Clare and Mick's to drop off an anniversary card. I didn't feel too good when we got home; I think it is something I've eaten.

Thursday 26th March

Mr Adam's called me into his office this morning to tell me that I have been chosen to be a prefect. I was dead chuffed! In Biology we had to snip a bit of bone to reveal our rat's vagina. I wasn't quite sure where I was meant to cut.

Tuesday 31st March

I had to get up dead early so I could go to school to go off with the rest of the cast and crew of West Side Story to see Starlight Express in London. It was all done on roller-skates and it was fantastic and I really enjoyed it. Poor old Andrew couldn't go because he was poorly.

Wednesday 1ˢᵗ April

Mrs Beer took a minibus full of our biology group to Birmingham University to listen to three lectures. I went to one on transplantation, one called 'Green Medicine', and one on cancer. The first one was the most interesting. We had a great laugh and Mrs Beer said she would take us on a field trip somewhere.

Thursday 2ⁿᵈ April

School was a good laugh today as it was our election. I voted Conservative and helped organise the polling booth and count the votes. In Biology, I cut into the thoracic cavity of my rat. I was very pleased with myself that I had managed to do it. I got my prefect badge today!

Friday 3ʳᵈ April

I had a mock driving test today but failed. At least I now know what I need to improve on! We had a family evening in, after Andrew and I had walked the dogs.

Sunday 5ᵗʰ April

We all went to church, which was amazing. The service was boring but, during communion, a church mouse came out for a run and I laughed my head off, because he was so cute.

Wednesday 8th April
School was good, except I don't really like starting the day off with rat dissection. It's a bit too near breakfast. After school, Granddad was at home as he had been to see a production at Rob's school in the afternoon. We went to see it in the evening. Granddad is staying the night and he showed me his map of Crete, where he is planning to go on holiday.

Thursday 9th April
Election Day
I finished my rat dissection today, which was a great relief. I spent three lessons on it. I took the rat home to show Mum and Dad! I stayed up until midnight, listening to some of the election results. It looks as if it will be really close.

Tuesday 21st April
Andy's 16th Birthday
Granddad came with his walking pal and they went off for a walk with their backpacks. They are so funny. We had a late tea as Andy and Dad had gone to play golf. Sam has come up to sit on my bed. He is so cute!

Thursday 23rd April
Jonathan and Paula came at 9.30 am and all of us (apart from Robert) went off to Manchester to see 'Les Miserables'.

We walked round Manchester for a while and then had a lovely lunch. The show was three hours long, and it was brilliant. We all really enjoyed it. Jonathan and Paula came back for tea and then went home.

Thursday 30th April

I wasn't allowed anything to eat or drink for breakfast. I went to school so I could have my English and Chemistry lessons. Mum collected me and we borrowed Judy's video camera and then went to Stafford. Dr Gibson videoed the gastroscopy. It was OK but I didn't feel too good afterwards. We watched the film when I got home. It was brilliant and very, very interesting. I'm tired now and looking forward to a good night's sleep.

Sunday 10th May

I woke up and realised that I had started my periods. About time too!

Friday 5th June

I had a driving lesson this morning at 7.30 am, and I had my test at 8.40 am. I failed. The weather was dreadful and it was really, really busy. I was upset all day. Mum collected me from school early and went down to give blood, but didn't feel too good. Dad also gave blood and he fainted and went really sweaty.

Thursday 2ⁿᵈ July
It was Mrs Broad's last day as she is leaving to have a baby.
We gave her the hippopotamus that we had bought for her
and she was really pleased. I had a great swim at lunchtime
and did 40 lengths.

Tuesday 7ᵗʰ July
John Hicks picked me up at 8.15am and I had my driving
test at 9.30 am. I had to do a turn in the road and reverse
round a corner. I PASSED! I was over the moon! Carole
bought me a road atlas, which is brill. After tea, I went for a
drive all on my own to Lichfield, which was great fun!

Friday 17ᵗʰ July
I got up at 2.30 am and went to school to go in the minibus
to Guernsey. We got there at about 3.30 pm. We put our
tents up and, after we had been down the pub, were all really
knackered, so we all slept well.

Sunday 19ᵗʰ July
It was our form's duty day today, so we had to do the
evening meal. We did coq au vin, which was mega doing it
for 120 people. It took us ages to clear up afterwards. We
then had a staff meeting, which was a laugh. Mr Martin is
a great bloke. It's really weird calling all the teachers by their
Christian names.

Tuesday 21ˢᵗ July
Today I went off for a tour of the island with Pat and Pete (Mrs Burrows and Mr Collinge). I had a nice sunbathe on a grassy bank and then went for a swim. In the evening we had lasagne prepared by Anne Parton's group. We then had a floating disco, which was ACE!

Thursday 27ᵗʰ August
It was Andrew's GCSE results today. He got 3As, 4Bs and a C. Well done him!

Thursday 3ʳᵈ September
I met Dad in Tamworth at lunchtime and then walked back to his office with him and then drove home. Later on, Mum and Dad took the dogs to be put down. After much discussion, we came to the conclusion that had to be done as they had caused us much heartache. Everyone was very upset.

The dogs had been causing us increasing problems, as they were prone to attacking other dogs and biting anyone who got in the way. After one particularly distressing incident, we felt that they had finally overstepped the mark.

Friday 4ᵗʰ September
Dad got me up early and I was at work at Boots at 8.30

am. I couldn't stop thinking about Sam and Lucky, and had to stop myself from crying. Mum collected me from work and I didn't do much in the afternoon. After tea, we had a game of cards. Dad won for a change!

Wednesday 9th September
I only had one lesson today, and that was Biology. Mr Tyler was really funny and sperm counts were a topic of conversation. He told us that an 18-year-old lad was capable of ejaculating seventeen times a day. WOW! No wonder all they want is sex at that age!

Friday 25th September
In the evening it was the Harvest Supper and Dad was in charge of the entertainment. They did 'Mr Bean goes to church' and 'Mr Bean becomes churchwarden'. Peter was Mr Bean and Dad was the vicar, with a hideous wig on. It was so funny.

Wednesday 7th October
My 18th Birthday
Dad took me to school so I could have my early morning swim. I had loads of cuddles from friends and, after my second swim at lunchtime; my 'friends' nicked all my clothes and put a condom filled with water in my shoe. I had to go looking for my clothes with just a towel wrapped round me! After school,

I had loads of presents including a sewing machine from Mum and Dad, and a necklace from Dad that he had designed. It's a rainbow over the top of a heart opal. It's beautiful! We went out for a meal and Jonathan and Paula came, which was a lovely surprise.

Sally was now eighteen and busy applying to universities with a view to doing a teaching degree, but, yet again, her health challenges continued with a bout of shingles. Note, however, that she doesn't have a few days off and take to her bed.

Monday 26th October
Mum and I went off early by train to Liverpool and the Institute of Higher Education. We had a guided tour and it is a great place. We also had a lovely look round Liverpool, and I bought a personal stereo with the money that Grandma had given me for my birthday.

Tuesday 27th October
I had a very slow start today and went to the doctor, who confirmed that I do have shingles. It is very painful and itchy. However, I still felt OK so I went in to work at Boots. I wish I hadn't though, because I felt knackered afterwards. I didn't do much in the evening, as I was really uncomfortable. It's all blistery and yuck.

Thursday 29th October

Mum, Robert and I went off to Nottingham today to visit the polytechnic and also meet up with Sue and Emma. We had lunch at Sue's house and then Mum and me went to the polytechnic, which is lovely, especially the science department. I didn't feel too good in the evening. My shingles is getting on my nerves.

Sunday 1st November

I had a lovely lie in this morning and then did some homework. I phoned Jonathan Dudley, and he has fixed up the tickets for 'Miss Saigon' in London. Brill or what!

Monday 2nd November

I went to school for a half day today. Everyone wanted to keep away from me because of my shingles. They don't believe that you can't catch it! I went to sleep in the afternoon and then went to the doctors for more tablets and cream. I'm not really sure what to do about school, as I don't really feel 100%.

Thursday 5th November

I went to see Dr Gibson today, and also his house doctor, Hamish Duncan, who is lovely. I had a mega blood test and I have to come back in ten days for another one.

Saturday 7th November
I didn't go to work today because of my shingles. I keep getting very tired. I didn't feel like eating and in the evening I was sick. I got hardly any sleep. It was either one end or the other!

Sunday 8th November
I spent all day in bed with Mum, as we both have sickness and diarrhoea.

Friday 13th November
School was OK. It was Marcus's birthday so the lads taped him to a chair and carried him into the playground, where they covered him in stink bombs. They are cruel!

Sunday 15th November
I went to church today as I was serving. I did some homework in the afternoon, and then, after tea, we had a silly half an hour tickling each other, which was great immature fun!! Everyone's a child at heart!

Sunday 22nd November
I was suffering from depression for not having a man! I had a lovely chat to Andrew, which was very brotherly/sisterly.

Monday 23rd November

I really wanted to speak to Dave today, but I thought it best to get to know him better first. After school, I watched Channel Four's 'Big Breakfast' that we had recorded this morning. Every week they feature a different family, and this week it is Robert, Caroline, Jonathan, Kathryn, and Timothy Ellis. It's so funny!

Friday 27th November

After school, I watched 'Big Breakfast' from this morning. They featured the photo that we had sent in of Robert Ellis in drag at a harvest supper concert. It was so funny!

Sunday 29th November

Tina came over and we had a revision session. We then decided to go to the cinema and Tina drove. On the way back, we had a crash when a twat of a bloke didn't look and came out of a side road and hit us in the middle of the car. It was dreadful and I have got whiplash. Tina is fine. We were very lucky.

Monday 30th November

Dad took me into school and I had lots of questions about my neck collar, and loads of sympathy. I went back to school later on for a parent's evening. Tina and I had to dissect a rat! Thank you Mrs Beer and Mr Tyler very much!

Friday 4th December

School was just a complete laugh today. It was the last day before out exams start, so we made a grotto in the sixth form centre and the lads invited the first years in. Dave, the sexy beast, was Santa! Mum gave me a Shiatsu massage in the evening, which was very nice, but it would have been better if Dave could have done it!

Thursday 17th December

I had a lovely lie in and then went into school for my last exam; general studies. In the evening we went to Harper's Night Club. We arrived at 9.30 pm and danced the night away until 2.15 am. I wore my new red dress. We eventually got to bed at about 3.45 am and I stayed at Rachel's. It was an excellent night and everyone was great. Unfortunately, Dave got off with someone else.

Wednesday 23rd December

I had a little lie in and then Judy took me into work at Boots from 12.00 till 5.00. Dad collected me and I had a relaxing evening in while Mum and Dad went to Peter and Ruth's. I had a lovely letter and card from Dr Fairbrother today from Mansfield.

Friday 25ᵗʰ December
I had loads of presents and Mum and Dad were quite taken aback with their 'Miss Saigon' tickets that Jonathan Dudley had organised. We watched 'Shirley Valentine' on TV later on.

Tuesday 29ᵗʰ December
I had a lovely lie in today and didn't wake up until 10.00 am. In the afternoon, Dad and I did a bit of planning for our New Year's Party, including thinking of silly names for everyone.

Thursday 31ˢᵗ December
I worked at Boots from 10.00 till 4.00 and it was really busy. In the evening we had our party with the Grews and Hollidays, Judy's mum, dad and sister's family. We had some brilliant games and we all had a great time. We had a good dance and made a lot of noise. I went to bed at 3.30 am.

CHAPTER TEN

THERE'S MORE TO LIFE THAN EXAMS

1993

Not a great start to 1993.

Friday 1ˢᵗ January
Clare and Mick came at 10.30 am and we went off to the dry ski slope at Swadlincote. Clare didn't ski as she is really big now as she is pregnant. I fell awkwardly and dislocated my thumb. They took me to the hospital to have it pulled back into place. It hurt a lot afterwards, even after a local anaesthetic. What a start to the New Year. It's really awkward doing anything without the use of your thumb.

Saturday 2ⁿᵈ January
My thumb is twice the size this morning and my thumb is very painful. Clare and Mick came to see me and stayed for a couple of hours.

Sunday 3rd January
We all went to church for Peter's last family service today. It will be bad next week as it is his last service. My thumb has throbbed for most of the day. Robert spent a bit of time tickling my feet, which was nice.

Monday 4th January
Mum took me to Burton Hospital to see a doctor about my hand. He was a right twat, sarcastic and very unsympathetic. He also said that I might have to have an operation. My hand is now in plaster and feels very heavy.

Tuesday 5th January
School was dreadful as I had all my mock results and I got all 'U's. I was so disappointed. Mum has had a busy day as she went with Ruth to help with her curtains at Stratford vicarage. Mum and Dad went to a PCC meeting in the evening, so they were stressed out when they got home!

Thursday 7th January
Mum and I went on the train to West Hill College for my interview. We had various talks and then my interview was at 11.30 am. I thought it went really well.

Sunday 10th January
PETER'S LAST SERVICE
It was really sad this morning and I cried loads. I shall really miss Peter's love and support. My thumb is still hurting and getting on my nerves and I'm nervous about my interview tomorrow.

Monday 11th January
Dad took me to Scarborough's North Riding College where I had an interview. It's a nice place and we had a walk down by the sea. The only problem is distance (145 miles), and getting my 'A' level results.

Tuesday 12th January
I was woken up by a terrible pain in the lower part of my tummy, it was dreadful. I went into school but I didn't feel very well. I had loads of different emotions inside, painful thumb and tummy and worrying what was causing it but my biggest pain is that Peter and his family are moving on Thursday.

Wednesday 13th January
Mum and I got up early and caught the 7.15 am train to York. I had an interview at the York and Ripon College. The bloke who interviewed me was a headmaster. I don't think that headmasters should interview you. I wasn't very confident, as I didn't like the look of him.

Monday 18th January

Mum took me to Manchester Polytechnic for an interview today, and it went very well, even though we were not that impressed with the place. Robert has enjoyed his birthday, and the Grews and the Ellises came to see him after school. Mum and Dad went off to their yoga class later on, and I phoned Jonathan and Paula to fix up arrangements for Saturday. I can't wait.

Saturday 23rd January

Mum and Dad went off to Leamington to Jonathan and Paula's and then off to see 'Miss Saigon' in London. Rob and I went on the train to Leamington. We had a little shop and then went to Jonathan's house for the afternoon. We waited for Mum and Dad, who had a lovely surprise to see us. We had some tea and a chat and got home late. They had all enjoyed the show and I am so pleased I bought Mum and Dad that present.

Sunday 24th January

I forgot to put yesterday that, not last night but the night before, I had a really good dream about Dave that we fell in love; but it was only a dream. I went to church. It was OK, but not the same without Peter.

Thursday 28th January

I went to school to do my chemistry practical assessment and then Mum picked me up and we went for my interview at Derby University. I was pleased with how it went. At 5.30 pm we caught the coach from church to go to Peter's induction at Stratford. It was all very ceremonial. There was a nice reception afterwards and Jonathan and Paula were there too.

Saturday 30th January

I went to town with Mum and bought a book by Dr Manny Patel (a yoga teacher) for Dad's birthday. In the evening, Robert, Caroline, Kathryn, Jonathan, and Timothy came. We had a Chinese meal and had a great time.

Monday 1st February

Mum collected me from school and we went to Burton Hospital to have my plaster taken off. It was great to have my arm free again.

Wednesday 3rd February

Dad and I went to Liverpool Institute of Higher Education today. I had a good interview and look around. I did some of the motorway driving coming back.

Thursday 4th February

School was good today, except that Mrs Broad gave us loads of homework. I had a swim at lunchtime which was brilliant.

After school, Robert had Steph back to play. Young love!! I did a bit of homework but mainly we talked about loads of things and had a great laugh.

Thursday 11th February
I had a chemistry lesson and then went off for occupational therapy on my thumb. I swam at lunchtime and then came home. I fetched Andy after his 'Guys and Dolls' practice. He was in an ace mood as he had just got off with a girl at school. They had bought each other Valentine's cards. Andy is besotted with her but he will miss her this week as she is off to Tenerife on holiday.

Thursday 18th February
I had a fantastic time at Harper's Night Club. Dave bought me a drink and Julie and I danced with him all night. Unfortunately, I didn't get the last dance with him. Also today, Clare has had a little girl, Megan Emily.

Friday 19th February
Mum and I went to see Clare and Megan. She is beautiful. I went to Dave's party at 8.00 pm.

Tuesday 9th March
It was the dress rehearsal for 'Guys and Dolls' today. I am a prompt and have to wear a headset, and also direct the scene changes.

Wednesday 10th March
I had a swim in the afternoon, and then Andy and I had a little rest after school before setting off for the premiere of 'Guys and Dolls'. Andy was playing the part of Sky Masterson. It went really well and I didn't have to do any prompting.

Saturday 13th March
I worked at Boots from 10.00 till 4.00 and then watched the evening performance from the audience. Andy and me went to the party afterwards and had a great time.

Wednesday 24th March
I went to school early for a swim and did 50 lengths in 25 minutes! In the afternoon I had an appointment with my gynaecologist and Tina went with me for moral support. He explained that I couldn't go on the pill because of my liver problems, so there is no way to make my periods more regular. It also means that my methods of contraception are limited. What a downer. I felt a bit depressed. Why can't my body function like everyone else's?

Friday 26th March
School was ace today. Mark and Jason were such good fun in Biology, and then in Chemistry, we had a water fight and I got soaked. I had to take my shirt off and borrow Andy's jumper. The lads were teasing me, saying that I looked like a barmaid.

Tuesday 27th April

I didn't feel too well at school today. In General Studies, we had a discussion that upset me so much that I nearly had to walk out. It was about fatal diseases and death. I had a lie down after school, as I didn't feel 100%.

Wednesday 28th April

I went to school for the morning and then went off to Stafford for a blood test. I passed out afterwards, which caused quite a disturbance.

Friday 21st May

Last ever day at school.

Mr Tyler was most amused by our gift of a sex book for the over 30s. We all went down to the pub at lunchtime, including the teachers.

Wednesday 26th May

I got up early and went for a swim. I did 100 metres in 1 minute 41 seconds. Mum and I went into Sutton later on and tried on a ball gown. It looked ace, but I had no intention of buying it. In the evening, Mum found an old diary of hers and we had a good giggle. Mum then gave me a massage, which was lovely.

Thursday 27th May

There has been a reshuffle of John Major's cabinet today. Kenneth Clarke is the new chancellor, instead of Norman Lamont.

Saturday 29th May

I worked at Boots from 11.30 to 5.30, and it was really busy. Later on I dressed up as a St Trinian and went on a pub-crawl with the rest of the Boots girls to raise money for Cancer Research. Loads of lads kept trying to lift my skirt to undo my suspenders. Randy sods!

Sunday 6th June

I did revision all morning; it was a real scorcher of a day. In the afternoon, we set off to Baxterly for Megan's christening. I was a godparent along with Clare's cousin and fiancé, Richard and Nathalie. We had a great get together afterwards.

Monday 7th June

I was a bit of a nervous wreck today as it is the start of my 'A' levels. Chemistry today, Biology on Thursday and Chemistry again on Friday.

Wednesday 16th June
MY LAST EXAM
The exam wasn't as bad as I thought it would be, so I have

now finished school FOREVER. I came home to tidy my room and have a bit of a move round. Mum and I went to see 'Indecent Proposal' at the cinema. It was excellent.

Monday 5th July

I rang Eric this morning. The reason we have not seen them for so long is that he and Janette have separated, and he is living in Burton. This upset me and I have arranged to see him tomorrow. Mum and Dad don't know that though. I want to reunite Eric and Emma on my own and Mum would want to see him and I wouldn't be able to get a word in edgeways.

Tuesday 6th July

I met up with Eric in Rugeley and we had a good chat about Emma and his separation. He has been living on his own since last August. I really must get in touch with Emma now.

Monday 12th July

I went swimming first thing, which was invigorating. I did some chores and then collected Elizabeth and looked after her until Judy came. I also babysat for the Grews in the evening. I watched a controversial adaptation of a book by D H Lawrence called 'The Rainbow'.

Wednesday 14th July

I went swimming first thing and then went home to start making a blouse. I looked after Elizabeth all afternoon. In the evening, Grandma and Granddad came over and we all went to see Andrew in a show at school called 'Curtain Call'. It was brilliant and was a mixture of dance and musicals. Andy sang songs from Blood Brothers, Miss Saigon and Grease.

Sunday 18th July

I slept in until late morning and then got up and made a quiche and a cake. In the evening, we all went to a centenary service at Wilnecote Congregational Church and Dad was presented with a picture for his long service as church treasurer.

Wednesday 21st July

I went to school at midday and we loaded up the coaches to travel to Poole, to catch the ferry to Guernsey. I am in Mr Martin's group along with other 6th formers. It is now 10.40 in the evening and it's really nice sitting out on deck having a laugh.

Thursday 22nd July

We docked at 6.00 am and we are all exhausted. I spent most of the day on the beach, as it is very hot. We played football later on and Stuart knocked my glasses off. He was very apologetic. Bless him!

Friday 23rd July
We went off to St Peter Port and I bought a bargain camera from Boots. We had a floating disco in the evening, which was OK, but the sea was a bit choppy.

Saturday 31st July
I got up early as I was on duty with Graham and Shirley Martin. We had to use up all the leftovers and later on the tents came down. It was a lovely day and I did some sunbathing and then packed my bag in the open air! We went to the pub later on and then, slept in a marquee, which was a laugh.

Sunday 1st August
We got up early and were taken to St Peter Port to board the ferry home. We had a superb crossing and it was great out on deck. We arrived home at 1.00 pm and it was great sleeping in my own bed.

Monday 2nd August
I had a great lie in, and then it was a case of washing, ironing and packing, ready for Tenerife.

Wednesday 4th August
We had a lovely first day in Tenerife. I swam 20 lengths before breakfast. We then sunbathed by the pool. Andy and I went to see a hypnotist in the evening. He was superb.

Friday 6th August

We met a lovely family today. Wendy and Roger and Mark, who is my age, and Lindsey who is 16. We had a game of water polo together. We had a great laugh with them.

Sunday 15th August

We met up with the Pettits again for sunbathing and swimming. We also went out for a meal with them, which was a good giggle. Andy sang in the karaoke later on, and Lindsey and I were his backing group. We have loads in common with the Pettits; it's really funny.

Tuesday 17th August

We had a long day by the pool, getting as much sun as possible, and then waved the Pettits off. Our flight was at 10.00 pm so we didn't get home until 4.30am!

Wednesday 18th August

We all slept until late and then Mum and I went round to see Judy. At 2.30 pm, Mum and Dad had to go to an emergency PCC meeting to meet the possible new vicar. I'm missing the Pettits and very worried about tomorrow.

Thursday 19th August

I had a really crap day today as I got my exam results; All 'U's. There's more to life than exams.

Friday 20th August
I went to the careers office and they were very helpful. The highlight of the day was when I went to see Clare, Mick, and Megan. I needed that cuddle from her!

Monday 23rd August
Eric came with Alex and took Rob off to play golf. In the afternoon I went with Mum to have a look around the job centre and, also to the careers office for more information. Dr Gibson phoned later on and said that he will try to find out if I would pass a nursing medical.

Saturday 28th August
I worked at Boots from 10.00 till 4.00 and then Dad picked me up. Dad was in a really ace mood. He and I have a thing about names. In fact I think he's getting a bit worried that I'm getting obsessed with them.

Tuesday 7th September
I went to enrol on a pre-nursing course at Tamworth College, so I will be starting soon; excellent! I saw Natalie later on and had a lovely chat.

Wednesday 8th September
Dad took me to Stafford for a gastroscopy, which went well. Dr Gibson looked different. I don't know why; he just did. I went to sleep in the afternoon.

Monday 13th September
Andrew had his driving test this morning and failed. He was quite annoyed. I had an appointment at the DHSS to see if I can get income support, but I probably cannot. Stupid system! Dad was in a daft mood later on, so we had a \good laugh in the evening.

Friday 17th September
I had the morning to myself so I did my nursing application. I went to see Mr Martin and asked if he would write a reference for me. I then brought Andrew home. He has gone out to a party tonight and I am stuck with babysitting.

Sunday 18th September
I really wished I had a boyfriend. I don't know why I wrote that.

Monday 20th September
I started the Access course at Tamworth College today. We seemed to spend far too much time messing about, trying to sort out the timetable.

Tuesday 21st September
Dad took me to Tamworth and I worked in the college library for a little while before I had a lesson. We then had three hours of maths, which was pathetic. I was really bored. After tea, I went round to see Judy and had a lovely chat with her.

Sally was going through one of the unhappiest periods of her life. She had failed her 'A' levels, many of her friends had gone off to college or university, she was having great difficulty getting to do what she really wanted to do, she had no boyfriend, and her relentless health problems continued. Her natural cheerfulness and optimism were being tested to the limit. Where would she get the inspiration to persevere?

Saturday 25th September
I worked at Boots from 10.00 till 4.00, which was OK ish. I feel a bit depressed and unfulfilled in various different ways. I really wish that I could go straight into a nursing career now.

Wednesday 29th September
College was crap today and I don't think that I am going to continue with the course. I had a letter from Eric today. He has written to Emma, so I am really pleased with myself.

Monday 18th October
I felt yuck today so I didn't go into college. Dr Abbott thinks that I have a water infection, so I have to drink loads (which means wee loads too!!)

Saturday 23rd October

I went with Mum and Dad to a yoga seminar at Bilston, run by the Life Foundation. It was so incredible that I cannot put it into words. Manny Patel is so lovely, I could listen to him forever, and Annie's movements are so beautiful. I felt so good after a wonderful day, and had so much fun too.

Friday 29th October

I went with Mum and Dad to Mansfield today and we had a good shop. We then went to the hospital to see Mr Fairbrother who showed us round. We went to Manvers Ward and saw some of the nurses that nursed me. It was lovely to see him again. He is such a caring and gentle man.

Thursday 4th November

I had to see Dr Gibson today, except I saw some other doctor, which pissed me off. I have got to increase my drug dose. I'm pissed off with my life.

Tuesday 9th November

When I came back from college I made the decision to give up the course. I phoned the Voluntary Health Service and I have an appointment next week.

Tuesday 16th November

I had an interview with the voluntary services, so, hopefully, I will be given a placement soon.

Sunday 21st November

I got up really early and went with Mum and Dad to their yoga course at Bilston. It was brilliant. I joined in with a workshop in a small group. Johti talked to me about diet and nutrition and I have learnt some interesting things, so I am considering eating much more vegetarian meals. At the end we sang a lovely song and all held hands. I sat next to Kevin who was quite a card. He was very chatty, and admired my blonde hair. He gave me a piece of chewing gum, as that was all he had to give me.

Saturday 4th December

I worked at Boots from 10.00 till 4.00, and then met up with Sarah and Juliette. We went to Carole's house as she was celebrating being licensed as a lay reader in the cathedral today. In the evening I babysat at Judy's for five girls; all the Grews, Juliette, and Rebecca. Chaos!

Wednesday 15th December

I went off to Manchester with Ruth to see The Phantom of the Opera. It was excellent! The music means much more now. The phantom was incredible in his make-up and mask, and he really made me jump when he came crashing down onto the stage; amazing.

Thursday 16th December

Ruth and I had a lie in and then went to Lichfield, where Ruth caught a bus home. I went to see Dr Gibson in the afternoon and I have lost half a stone. I had a blood test and my previous test results showed an improvement.

Friday 17th December

I had a phone call from St Michael's Hospital saying that I have got an interview for a position of ancillary help!! Eric also phoned to say that he saw Emma on Tuesday, so I am really chuffed that I have got them back together.

Tuesday 21st December

I had my interview at St Michael's Hospital for a part-time ancillary job. The interview went well, but I didn't get the job. I think that it wouldn't have been that suitable, as it was only two hours a day.

Tuesday 28th December

It is snowing a little, but the Pettits still came. We all had a ride up to the golf club for a drink before lunch. After lunch the lads had a game of snooker and I had a great laugh with Lindsey. We then all had a game of Pictionary, and the Pettits went home at 8.00 pm. We have had a lovely day.

Friday 31st December

Dad went off to work, and I went with Rob and Mum to do a little 'sales' shopping. We went to see 'Jurassic Park' in the afternoon and then to a New Year's party at Carole's in the evening. This was a good laugh.

CHAPTER ELEVEN

A BIG DECISION

07/01/1994

I got up late. Mum was at work. I did chores, such as ironing etc. Mum got back for lunch. The afternoon flew by. Mum and I made a trinket box out of plastic canvas; it looks lovely. Dad made me laugh later on.

Little did we know in January 1994 what a challenging and life-changing year it would turn out to be. Sally was keeping busy with a part-time job at Boot's the chemists, babysitting for friends, doing lots of creative crafts, keeping in touch with her friends and trying to plan her career. It was becoming increasingly obvious that her liver was struggling, as her energy level was not sustainable for long. As a consequence the hospital visits intensified. She had always enjoyed close personal relationships with her various consultants but did not suffer what she saw as incompetent stand-ins gladly.

10/02/1994

I had an appointment with Doctor Gibson today, except I didn't see him. I saw another twatty doctor instead. He was really incompetent. I was very annoyed.

Sally was always very determined to do something once it was in her head. She wanted to visit her friend Ruth at Hull University and despite bad weather was intent on going.

14/02/1994

I had a restful day today. I made a heart cake. It was bitterly cold today. It is forecasting snow tonight and tomorrow. Shit! I was hoping to go to see Ruth in Hull.

15/02/1994

There was loads of snow this morning. Dad didn't really want me to go to Hull but I did and there were no delays. I got here at about 2.15 pm. Ruth met me. We had an excellent time in the evening. We met all Ruth's pals; Richard, Ali, Tall Dave, Big Dave, John, Julie, and last, but certainly not least, THOMAS!! He is lovely.

21/02/1994

Mum had the morning off work, as I wasn't too good. Later we went to town to pick up my photos, which are great, especially the one of Thomas and me. I have sent them to Ruth with a letter. I have felt up and down all day, so hopefully I will feel better tomorrow.

22/02/1994

I coughed up some blood this morning. At 11.00 am I went to see Doctor Deb. He said that I should go to see Doctor Gibson so at 12 I was there. Doctor Gibson doesn't really know what is wrong. I had a chest x-ray, blood test and chest scan but they won't be able to see if the scan is clear until I have another part of the scan next week. I feel pretty rotten.

23/02/1994

I felt dreadful today. We have had loads of snow so everyone was at home. Mum phoned Doctor Gibson, who said that I should come into hospital, so an ambulance fetched me.

The ambulance actually got stuck in the snow and it took all of our efforts to push the vehicle, with Sally inside it, off the drive.

24/02/1994

I had a crap night's sleep; in fact I don't think I slept at all. I was also in a lot of pain and I wasn't allowed any painkillers. Doctor Gibson came to see me first thing, bless him, he was lovely. Then at 3.20 pm I had an ultrasound with a full bladder. Apparently, I've got a bit of a spleen growth. Weird man! I also had an abdominal x-ray. Dad and Andy came in later; they stayed for ages.

26/02/1994

I was woken up in the middle of the night, which was a bit of a bugger. Then at 5.35 am it was thermometer time. At about 3.00 pm Clare, Mike and Megan came to see me, which was lovely. They stayed until about 5.15 pm. Then, after tea, Mum and Dad came. They stayed until about 9.15 pm. Dad was in a really giggly mood. When they had gone I phoned Andy.

27/02/1994

It was the usual routine this morning, being woken up at some ungodly hour. Mum came in after lunch and then Judy came – she stayed for quite a while. At about 7.15 pm Andy arrived. He stayed until about 9.30 pm. I have got quite bad tummy ache tonight.

28/02/1994

It was a normal sort of hospital day. Dr Gibson came to see me with a whole troop of doctors. I was woken up with my injection of Heparin. Mum and Granddad came to see me later but no one came at night as it was the induction service.

This related to the induction of our new priest-in-charge; Rev John Allan. The doctors were clearly struggling to find out what the problem was, but why isn't a CAT scan used as a first resort rather then last resort?

04/03/1994

I didn't get a good night's sleep and I felt rather dreadful with the pain going on and off all day. Peter Holliday came to see me at about 12.30 pm, which was lovely. Mum arrived and stayed until 8 ish. Doctor Gibson came to see me later and he still doesn't understand what is giving me the pain so I have to go for a CAT scan on either Monday or Tuesday.

06/03/1994

I woke up with dreadful pain in the early hours. I was given some pethidine. Doctor Fisher saw me a bit later and put me on a drip. He took some of the infected fluid off my tummy, which wasn't very nice. Doctor Gibson and a surgeon saw me later as they weren't sure if they were going to have to operate. Felt bloody awful

More tests followed over the next few days, accompanied by a lot more anxiety all round. Mum was about to take over the writing of the diary.

10/03/1994

Morning was just boring. Judy came. Audrey came later. Doctor Gibson saw me, and then Jonathon and Paula and all my family came. I didn't want Mum and Dad to go.

The following morning Sally had deteriorated further and the decision was taken to transfer her to the Queen Elizabeth Hospital, Birmingham. The ambulance took thirty-five minutes to make the journey from Stafford to Birmingham and Sally was taken to the intensive care liver ward. She was prepared for surgery, which was undertaken by David Mayer. Val had been at the hospital and so had accompanied her to Birmingham. I had a very brief message at the office to get myself over to the hospital. I was in such a state, but fortunately my very good friend Robert Ellis was around to accompany me to the hospital.

The CAT scan had revealed that a significant part of Sally's small intestines had been destroyed by infection. She was very seriously ill. We did not meet David Mayer until the next day, as he was exhausted after the late night operation, but another doctor explained what had happened and left us in no doubt how serious the situation was. Clearly all of Sally's fighting spirit was about to be put to the test once more. We could only pray that the combined forces of the doctor's skill, Sally's indomitable spirit and our love for her would pull her through.

The next day it was explained to us that a blood clot had blocked the small intestine, causing serious damage and necessitating the removal of 171 centimetres of the ileum, and the formation of a temporary ileostomy.

At this point Val took over Sally's diary.

12/03/1994

I am wired up to loads of machines and am very uncomfortable and hot. I have a bit missing from my insides (half of my small intestine) and a bit extra on the outside (ileostomy.) Robert Ellis brought Andy and Robert to see me but I was very dopey. I was looked after by Mark in the morning, Gus in the afternoon and Marie at night.

13/03/1994

Gave Mum a lovely hug when she came in at 8.00 am. Physio Helen is trying to get me to cough; must deep breathe and huff very regularly.

15/03/1994

Carole came in about 12.00. Doctor Gerry Somebody put a new Venflon in my arm. I had a scan on my legs. Lorraine took the catheter out and then the central line from my neck.

The stoma nurse came but I was asleep. Doctor Daniel Candidas (sexy Swiss surgeon) had a look at my ileostomy. Had an orange lolly. 4.00 pm used the commode. Doctor Candidas (with a team of nine doctors) told me my ileostomy could be reversed, maybe in six weeks. Moved to the ward.

16/03/1994
Used bathroom myself. Doctors said I could have free fluids. Judy came in with Robert, Mum, Peter Holliday and Carole. Went for a long walk down the corridor.

17/03/1994
Andy came in to visit and was here when they put a feeding tube in my nose.

18/03/1994
Didn't feel well today. My wound has gone septic, so they took twelve clips out and because it is now an open wound they packed it with Sorbison and dressed it. Dad watched this! [I was always the queasy one!] *My temperature is up and I feel very low and exhausted. Mum and Robert came on the train. Mum stayed to help get me ready for bed but one of the nurses turfed her out, which upset me. Anyway I found it made me cry so I suppose that means I am getting better, as earlier I was too weak to cry. Mum is staying.*
19/03/1994

Doctor Elwyn Elias came round and said that he had seen my notes for ten years but had never met me before. [He would be Sally's new consultant.] *Mum bought a birthday present for Elizabeth Grew. It was Bright Lights. We had a little go with it to check that it worked and then wrapped it up using micropore.*

20/03/1994

I had a bath, then had my dressing changed. Emma and Sue and Dad and Robert came. Jonathon and Paula also popped in whilst Mum and Dad were over at Nuffield House (residential accommodation for relatives of patients). Eric also came. I walked quite a bit and felt a lot better. I am still being fed by tube, 10 tins a day. Each tin has 250 calories. It's called Peptamen. Carnation makes it. I have put on weight.

21/03/1994

Andy came in on the train and Mum went home on the train. Daniel Candidas said I may have to have an angiogram later in the week. My temperature is still up so I am totally fed up – started my jigsaw.

23/03/1994

Mum, Dad and Andy went to Bath to have a look at the university. Judy came to be with me and she stayed all day to 6.00 pm. Mr McMasters came round and everyone was fussing round and standing to attention. Apparently he was the founder of the Liver Unit and is a surgeon. Peter Holliday popped in at 12.45 pm. Mum, Dad and Andy called in on their way back from Bath.

26/03/1994
Mum came in at 12.00 and we stayed on the ward quietly. We started to plan going somewhere but my stoma bag filled with blood again. This is not at all funny and I am worried and fed up. The doctors and nurses are all reassuring me that it's just a blip.

27/03/1994
Mum and Dad came in early and wheeled me down to the chapel for the Palm Sunday service. Back on the ward, Marie and Di and Robert and Caroline came to see me. Everyone on the ward was watching the football match at 5.00 pm, Aston Villa v Manchester United. Eventually Villa won. That should make Rob happy.

Sally's slow progress continued and she was eventually allowed home on the 31st March. The nurse came in daily to dress the wound. Our main concern was how much strain the operation had put on her liver.

25/04/1994

Dad took me to liver clinic and I saw Mr Mayer and Daniel (sexy) Candidas. Mr Mayer said that my bilirubin level is still too high to think about a reversal of the stoma and the current level means that it is time to think about transplanting. That worried me. Hopefully, the bilirubin level will drop - it had better! I'm so glad I saw Daniel. I also went to the ward and saw another yummy person – and that was Gus!

27/04/1994

Mum and Andy went to have a look at Bradford University, so I was on my own all day. The stoma nurse came and was pleased with how I was coping. I phoned the hospital to see what my bilirubin level was. It's gone up from 143 to 201 so I am a bit worried that Mr Mayer will want me to think about a transplant. Mum and Andy had a good day.

03/05/1994

The nurse (a different one again – Cheryl) came at 10.30 am and changed my dressing. It looks OK. I heard that Glenys Beveridge is improving and has had something to drink today, which is great news. I made a cake this morning. Robert had a friend for tea. My ileostomy was hurting, as something I've eaten doesn't agree with me. I think it's tomatoes.

09/05/1994

Dad took me to the liver clinic in the afternoon. We were early, so we went to find Abe. He was pleased to see me and gave me a kiss! Then we saw Mr Mayer. He wants to put off the reversal as long as possible until he can be sure that my liver is coping. One doctor said that a cirrhosed liver only lasts about 15 years. They were pleased with me anyway.

This was a real setback. Sally had been looking forward to being put together again and get rid of the tedium of having a stoma.

12/05/1994

I rang Mr Mayer's secretary to ask if he could ring me back and he did. In view of the high bilirubin level he wants to have me in for tests. I thought he would.

28/05/1994

After a bath and bag change, I went into work for the first time in ages, just for two and a half hours, so I could get back into it slowly. I really enjoyed it. I was knackered when I got back home so I had a sleep. Woolly invited me round to her house in the evening so I went. Sophie was there too. We had a pizza and a laugh.

Sally was admitted to the Queen Elizabeth Hospital on the 6th June for more blood tests and an angiogram.

She describes this procedure in great detail in her diary. She was also still able to see the funny side of things as well as being fascinated by medical procedures.

07/06/1994

I was moved to East 3 Liver Unit so I could be seen on the ward round. Simon (surgeon) kept making me laugh by winding up my humping dog (a wind up toy)!

08/06/1994

I was nil by mouth because of my angiogram. I had to have a Venflon installed and antibiotics to prevent any infection from the dye. I had a bit of an allergic reaction to one of the antibiotics. With the x-ray equipment they were able to guide the catheter in through my groin and up to my liver. I couldn't feel the catheter but the dye felt very warm when it was injected. I had to lie flat and keep my leg very still.

09/06/1994

Dominic said that the angiogram needed to be looked at very carefully by Doctors Elias, Mayer, and Buckels, so I am waiting. I had a special blood test called a split bilirubin, which apparently can tell where bile is coming from. Clever eh?

13/06/1994

I woke up at 4.00 am with a chronic pain in my left kidney. Mum and Dad took me back into the Queen Elizabeth. I eventually had 50mg of Pethidine, but it soon wore off so I had another dose. Later they gave me 100mg, which knocked me out for the night. The x-ray and ultrasound seem to point to a kidney stone.

14/06/1994

I was much better this morning – just a dull ache. Mum and Dad came in and we all had a chat to Dominic, Dr Elias, and Mr Mayer about the big choice we have got to make. Either a transplant soon or risk leaving it. We are all a bit shocked.

We all three came out of the consultation in a state of shock. I backtracked into the room to ask if there really was a choice. Didn't Sally have to go for the transplant? Mr Mayer made it very clear that the decision to go for transplantation was a positive and courageous step that only the patient could take.

15/06/1994

Dad came in so she was here when Dr Elias came round. I'm getting quite a lot of pain from the kidney stone but Simon reckons I will pass it in due course. I now have to sieve my wee! Dad and I together spoke with Janet, the chaplain. I've got a booklet about transplantation and I spoke to two transplant co-ordinators, which was helpful. Gus is on tonight. Excellent!

20/06/1994
We had our tea in the garden, then Mum, Dad, and I went to the Queen Elizabeth for a Liver Patients' Support Group meeting.

Sally would get very involved with this group post-transplant.

24/06/1994
We had a tremendous storm with giant hailstones and thunder and lightning. It was quite fantastic to watch. I had a chat with Mum and Dad about having a liver transplant. I see it as that I will be having one and I think that I have come to terms with it now.

25/06/1994
I managed to find a needle stuck in the carpet with my toe this morning and the point is still in. Ouch!

28/06/1994
I went to the Victoria Hospital and had an x-ray on my toe.

There is a quarter inch of needle embedded in my toe, so I was sent off to Stafford and the doctor I saw thought it best if I see an orthopaedic surgeon tomorrow as the needle is rather close to the bone. So, something to look forward to tomorrow!

29/06/1994

Andrew took me into Stafford and we saw the orthopaedic surgeon, who said that it needs a little surgery and I'm booked in for tomorrow. What a bugger! Anyway it needs to come out. When I got home I made some nice krispie cakes, which are really yummy. Dad phoned the Pettits later on to invite them to Forest Hills at the end of August. That should be a good laugh if they come.

30/06/1994

Dad took me in early to Stafford and I was first into theatre. I just had a local but it bloody well hurt having a local anaesthetic injected into your toe. Anyway, all quarter inch of the needle has been removed. Thank goodness!

01/07/1994

Mum and Dad took me into the Queen Elizabeth. We saw Doctor Elias and had a lovely chat. He answered all my questions and queries. I made the decision to go onto the waiting list for a new liver. Next week I will get my bleeper.

We told Robert later on and he was a bit upset. I went with Mum and Dad round to Judy's for cards and at the end of the evening we told them all too. It all went very well. Andrew has gone to his leaver's ball tonight.

02/07/1994

I got up at a reasonable time and had a bath with my foot over the side so as to not get the bandage wet! Andrew got in at 6.45 am after being up all night. He slept in all morning!

03/07/1994

We went to Grandma and Granddad's and Peter and Joan's to tell them I am going to have a transplant.

07/07/1994

We had a really intense day today as I went to the Queen Elizabeth with Andy, Mum and Dad. We spoke to Fiona, the transplant co-ordinator, a surgeon, physiotherapist, and dietician. They also took some blood. I have been given my bleep too and, apparently, I am the only A negative blood group on the list, so I won't be waiting very long. This came as a bit of a shock. Robert Ellis came over later, which was nice.

08/07/1994

Mum and Dad went into school with Rob to tell his tutor and Mr Firth, the headmaster. Later on Andy and I went in too. I had a nice chat with Mrs Broad. I had a lovely snooze after lunch, and then I went round to see Glenys to tell her the news. Dad picked Emma up from the station and brought her home.

10/07/1994
I fell asleep in the garden. I am really tired tonight. I got a bit upset — all this waiting is really hard.

Sally spent the next few days telling family and friends about being on the transplant list. I told our extended family after the service at the local church where we had worshipped since coming to Longdon. Sally was getting increasingly tired and jaundiced, her eyes were yellow and she was losing weight. She needed to take an afternoon nap most days. Every time the telephone rang our hearts were in our mouths. Then we had a call at home…

21/07/1994
I made a pair of boxer shorts for Dad today — they are ace! After that I had an afternoon nap. I popped into Rugeley for a quick shop. Whilst I was out there was chaos at home as Caroline, a transplant co-ordinator, rang to say they had got a donor liver. Half an hour later Caroline rang back to say it was not good enough. Mum went into panic mode and Dad came home a bit stunned. I missed all the drama. We went to McDonalds for some tea.

23/07/1994

I went to church. It was John Taylor, which was nice. After lunch and a rest, we all went to Robert and Caroline Ellis's for a barbeque, we had a thunderstorm so Robert cooked in the garage and we ate inside. Timothy (their youngest) is so unbelievably cute – he is really quite a card. We had a nice time.

27/07/1994

I had an early lunch and rest before going to the QE Liver Clinic. I saw Doctor Elias and Mr Freeman, a consultant anaesthetist. We had a nice chat with him. We seemed to do a lot of waiting around. They took eight vials of blood today (greedy lot!) Emma phoned from Portugal later on. It was lovely to hear from her.

28/07/1994

Mum, Dad and me set off to Bangor for the International Yoga Conference. We had a lovely evening meal and a fun session. I am really tired now, as I haven't had a sleep today.

29/07/1994

Mum and Dad went to the early yoga session, and then we had breakfast. I walked into Bangor. It was a lovely day. After lunch I was ready for a rest, and then I went to Robert Holden's laughter workshop, which was excellent. I bought one of his books, which Robert signed. He's lovely. After tea there was a ceilidh. I just did one dance.

30/07/1994
I had a bath while Mum and Dad went to the early session of yoga. After breakfast Mum and I went to a dolphin talk, which was very good. Later on, after lunch, and after I had a sleep, we spoke to Manny, and then we came home. We had tea at a Little Chef, which was yummy.

01/08/1994
I completed an anniversary card for Mum and Dad, but it's for next year! Nothing like planning in advance! I went to see Natalie as she is back from France. She wasn't in so I had a lovely chat to Margaret (Natalie's mum). She was really upset about my illness. I'm tired now.

02/08/1994
I went for a long walk with Natalie and Margaret. I have started an embroidery for Mum, but she doesn't know that I am doing it.

03/08/1994
I popped into Rugeley to get some threads so I can start an embroidery for Emma's birthday. It's a koala bear. I had my photos back through the post. Maz came for lunch, and then

I rested. Carole and Adam came for tea and stayed for most of the evening. I have done quite a lot of laughing tonight!

07/08/1994
We all went to church. It was Carole's last service. She was presented with a few bits including the embroidery that I had done of the church. It was a nice day. I had a lovely rest after lunch, then, for the rest of the day I mainly did embroidery. I suppose I'm becoming a bit boring, but I'm addicted!! I'm tired now.

Carole was a lay reader at church and, along with husband Jason, was moving from Longdon to Harrogate.

10/08/1994
Today Mum and I went over to Aunty Sue's mum's in Uttoxeter. Em was there and we had a little look around the town before going back for lunch and had a really lovely morning. I had a tape through the post today from the Life Foundation. They had recorded the tape especially for me, one evening last week when they were camping. It was very special; I was quite touched.

28/08/1994
We set off at 9.00 am to Bolton to see our friends the Pettits; Roger, Wendy, Lindsey, and Mark.

We had a lovely lunch, went to see where Mum and Dad would be spending the night, and went to see Roger's golf club, just to please the boys. After tea we had a game and did a lot of talking and laughing.

29/08/1994
After breakfast we all went ten-pin bowling, which was a real giggle. I got a strike! We had lunch at a little pub, and then Roger and Dad went for a game of golf, while the rest of us went for a walk. We are going to stay for another night.

Sally was getting increasingly tired and rather fed up with waiting for news. She still kept busy with her embroideries, cooking and other home activities.

06/09/1994
I had a bit of blood oozing from my stoma so I was a bit concerned. I phoned the hospital and Dave Mootimer phoned me back and said to come in to clinic tomorrow.

07/09/1994
Mum drove me into the QE so I could see Dr Elias. He reassured me that everything is fine. I had a nice chat with Julie, the staff nurse. Apparently, they were doing two transplants today; busy bees. I do hope mine is soon.

09/09/1994

I phoned the liver clinic this morning to see if they could put me in touch with patients who have had transplants. They gave me the number for a girl called Natalie, who is 19 and is coming to see me on Sunday.

11/09/1994

I made a fruit cake for the village produce show! Natalie came to see me. She had a transplant five years ago. She looks great and is getting married soon. At 8.00 pm, Fiona, from the QE, rang. They have a liver for me! It's now 10.10 pm and I'm at the QE with Mum and Dad. Poor old Andy and Rob are at home a bit worried. They should be operating at about 7.30 am!! My last ever night with a knackered, scarred, yuccy liver!!

Well, this was it. Sally was literally jumping for joy, and had every intention of seizing the opportunity of a new life, with a new liver. We hurriedly got ready. Val and I would be staying in accommodation provided by the hospital. It is late when we arrived at the hospital. Sally was in a side room on her own, and had to wait for a junior doctor to install a Venflon in her arm, ready for the operation in the morning. He actually made quite a hash of it, which was very distressing to our already frayed nerves.

We eventually left her to try to get some sleep, and set off to find our room. The main entrance doors were locked for security reasons so we had to make our way down into the basement to exit the hospital. We came across the cleaners' who had just mopped the floor, as Prince Charles was due to visit in a few days' time. There was, of course, a zero chance that he would get to see their sparkling clean floor in the basement, but they said we could not walk over it, and we had to find an alternative route. Little did they know how close I came to kicking over their bucket of suds out of total frustration.

We rested, but didn't really sleep, as we wanted to accompany Sally to theatre in the morning. Sally was very calm next morning, and we walked with her as she was wheeled to theatre. The nurses were very chatty and caring, and when David Mayer, her surgeon, arrived they sedated her and we left.

We could only pray that everything went well. We tried to catch up on our sleep, and had regular updates from Fiona, the transplant coordinator, as to how things were going. She said that the operating team had to proceed carefully and slowly to access the old liver.

The next bulletin was to say that the new liver was in and was working well. Wow! We didn't know whether to laugh or cry! We were eventually allowed to see Sally in the intensive care unit, but, of course, she was still heavily sedated. When she opened her eyes for the first time, we were thrilled to see that the awful yellow jaundiced look in her eyes had been replaced with a wonderful white. The miracle was beginning to unfold.

Val took over writing the diary to record the events of the next five days.

12/09/94

6.00 am Went back to Sally's room with Graham.

6.30 am Helped to bath Sally.

7.00 am Sally had injection to relax her.

7.45 am Graham and I accompany nurses Mary and Carol as Sally is wheeled down to Theatre 3.

8.00 am Stay with Sally in the anaesthetic room until David Mayer (surgeon) arrives. The liver had arrived at 6.30 am.

8.25 am Sally is given anaesthetic and slips into a peaceful sleep. We then phoned the boys and Granddad and a few close friends.

9.40 am Had canteen breakfast.

10.00 am Went back to our room to sleep.

11.00 am Fiona (transplant co-ordinator) came to say that

Sally was stable, but the team expected that it would take some time to access the old liver due to previous surgery. The liver is from Newcastle, so Graham asks if that means that she will now be a Geordie!

11.30 am Graham phones Andy while I chat with Lynn and pass on the embroidered cross that Sally had done for Janet, the hospital chaplain.

12.00 Went for a walk to clear our heads.

1.00 pm Fiona came to tell us that the new liver was in and working.

1.10 pm Peter Holliday came and had lunch with us.

3.00 pm Judy brought Andy and Rob in.

3.30 pm Graham, Andy, and Rob go to see Fiona. All is well and the operation is almost over.

4.15 pm Graham and I see David Mayer, who explains how the operation went and what to expect when we see her, which will be in about 30 minutes' time.

5.30 pm still waiting with Andy outside ICU.

5.35 pm Graham and I go in to see her. She is still sleeping, with a dummy in her mouth and tubes everywhere. Andrew came in. We don't like to see her like this, but we can see that everything is as well as can be expected.

6.00 pm had tea in the canteen as we were all very hungry.

6.30 pm we all went back to see her, going in in turn. Judy said that she looked beautiful.

We said goodbye to Judy and the lads in the car park, and then went back to see Sally one more time, before returning to our room for a bath and then bed.

13/09/94

Went in to see her at 6.45 am to find her still sleeping. Graham came at 8.00 am and Sally is now half awake and moving around a little too much for Nurse John's comfort. Sally acknowledged Graham when he said that Andrew and Robert Ellis were coming in later. Robert and the lads arrive at 10.30 am and Sally is looking a lot better. I must learn lip reading or sign language to understand what Sally is trying to tell us. She keeps asking what time it is.

Brother Rob came up and tickled Sally's hand and I am captain of the cold flannel. Eric came in at 12.00 and again at 3.30 pm. Uncle Peter and David came in at 1.00 pm. Sally acknowledged all visitors. The arterial line was taken out, and, later on, the ventilator. In the evening the nasogastric tube was taken out and the ileostomy bag changed. Rob and Andy came over again, after having a sleep in our room. They then left at 5.00 pm with Peter and David. We stayed while Sally had an ultrasound scan and Jill took over the night duty. Sally's tiny spleen showed up on the scan and the new liver seems fine.

14/09/94

We went in to see Sally at 7.00 am to find her sitting in a chair having a wash, so just in time with the new nighties. The doctors came round at 8.30 am and Rev'd John Allen at 11.00 am. Two different doctors tried to get a new Venflon in (five attempts, then gave up). Sally was not amused. Graham stayed with Sally for a long time while I went in pursuit of Prince Charles, who was opening a new ward today. Sally had catheter out and is trying to manage without oxygen. Andrew and Robert came in on the train.

15/09/94

Sally had both drains out (ouch!) Nikki the physio walked her a few steps along the corridor just as Grandma, Granddad, and Raymond Marriott came in. Peter and Ruth came in the evening, so that is four vicars not counting the hospital chaplain. Sally Ann looked after Sally in the morning, Fiona in the afternoon, and Nikki at night. Also saw Nurse Gus, Maxine and Pat the cleaner.

16/09/94

Went in to see Sally at 7.30 am. The dressings have now been removed and all looks very well. Dr Neil Fisher came in *to say that he had phoned Stafford Hospital and Sister Jarvis and everyone sent their love. Chris Hammersley and Andy came in and helped Sally move up to Ward 4. Brother Peter came in and had lunch with me. Graham and Rob came in at 5.00 pm and Judy and Sarah at 7.00 pm. Judy took Rob home and I went home for the night, while Graham stayed the night. Sally felt absolutely whacked tonight.*

Sally now felt well enough to take over the writing of her precious diary.

17/09/94

Dad stayed with me all morning and Robert, Caroline, and Kathryn brought Mum in later. Uncle Peter, Auntie Joan, and David and Amy came in at 5.00 pm. A drug overdose patient came into the bed next to me.

18/09/94

Dad spent time with me this morning; all seems quiet on a Sunday morning compared with a weekday. Rob and Andy arrived, and, later on, Auntie Sue, Emma and Uncle Eric. I gave Emma her birthday present; a Koala bear embroidery. Sue bought me some lovely pyjamas. Eric made me laugh with some of his police stories. I had a really nice afternoon.

19/09/94

Dr Neil Fisher did my biopsy at 12.30pm. It wasn't too bad, but I had to lie on my bed for six hours. The results show a small amount of rejection, but nothing to worry about. Judy popped in to see me and I had some great post.

21/09/94

I missed seeing Mum and Dad today, but Robert Ellis, Marie and Natalie called in. There is a chance I could be going home by the weekend.

23/09/94

It took six attempts to do my blood test this morning; not very funny. I can go home once they have given me my pills. It was great to get into my own bed.

24/09/94

The Lichfield Mercury photographer came to take some pictures for next week's paper. Had lots of visitors and several naps, but still found it a tiring day.

25/09/94

The Pettits came at midday and I had a good chat and giggle with Lindsey.

27/09/94

Mum took Andrew to town to get a few things as he is off to Bath University on Sunday. Before that, Mum walked me up to the shop, which was quite an achievement for me. I had a lovely sleep after lunch. I have done a lot of laughing tonight, which is excellent exercise for my tummy!!

28/09/94

Mum took me to the hospital this morning, and on the way we picked up several copies of the Lichfield Mercury. There are two pictures of me on the front page and a really good write up as well. We had a phone call from the Express and Star later, and they want to do the story as well.

29/09/94

The Express and Star photographer came to take my picture and later on I was on their front page. I had quite a busy day, as I went into town with Mum and saw Mr John and lots of the other staff at Boots.

02/10/94

ANDREW LEAVES HOME!

Mum and Dad took Andy to Bath with a very full carload. Emma came over to spend the day with me, which was really nice. Eric also came in the afternoon. Mum and Dad came back at 8.00 pm with some video of Andy's room. I bet he is out on the razzle at the moment!

03/10/94

I wrote to Andy this morning and then Mum took me into the hospital for my appointment with Mr Buckels. He is really quite funny. He reduced some of my pills, so I am now taking six in the morning and six at night.

Three weeks after the transplant!

04/10/94

I wrote quite a lot of letters today, and walked to the shop to post them. After tea I went to my sign language class, and it is really good.

05/10/94

I sent Natalie a small embroidered box as a wedding present. She came to see me the day before I went in for my transplant, and she had her transplant five years ago.

06/10/94

I went to my pottery class at Lichfield College today; it is brilliant. I am making a large vase and a cute candleholder.

07/10/94

MY 20th BIRTHDAY

I had a little fridge from Mum and Dad. It is ace and is sitting in my bedroom looking really cool! Andy rang at 3.00 pm and I had a lovely chat with him.

09/10/94

We all went to church this morning and everyone was pleased to see me. It was a lovely day so we had lunch in the garden.

10/10/94

I did a bit of ironing and then went to the hospital to see Mr McMaster. He said that my blood results were very good and they are pleased with my progress.

12/10/94

I popped round to see Glenys and, later on, Andy rang. Mum spotted an advert for a green Aga in the paper, and by 10.00 am they had bought it. Ace!

13/10/94

I drove myself to my pottery class. I had a super time as I had a go on the wheel, and actually made a pot! In the evening, Dad was in a really daft mood and we all had a really good giggle

We were all amazed how quickly Sally resumed her 'normal' activities and five weeks after her transplant went to Alton Towers! She had also made up her mind to take up a nursing career and, despite obstacles in her way, was determined to succeed.

16/10/94

We all went to Alton Towers as we had some free tickets. I went on loads of rides and watched the Nemesis- it's amazing.

19/10/94

I was up early today and caught a train to the QE to see a nursing officer about taking up nursing. She was quite helpful.

We were now six weeks post-transplant.

22/10/94

Mum and I went swimming this morning. It was brilliant. I did 15 lengths. Not bad for my first swim with my new liver!

Sally had made a remarkable recovery and seemed to have made her mind up about pursuing a nursing career. She set about sending for nursing college prospectuses, and then completing application forms.

05/12/94

I had an appointment at the QE today and saw Mr Buckels, and then Jacki, the procurement transplant coordinator. She was able to tell me a bit about the donor, so I can write a letter. She was a 36-year-old woman who had a massive brain haemorrhage and died very suddenly. She was married with a family. I went up to the ward and saw David Mayer in the corridor. I then went to the theatres and saw the gang who operated on me! They are such a lovely lot.

08/12/94

I went to my pottery class this morning and my fruit bowl looks really great. I then went to register at the DHSS. It wasn't too bad and I saw a job I quite fancied - theatre assistant at Little Aston Hospital - so they are going to send me an application form.

27/12/94

It was a very wet day so I completed my application form for the job at Little Aston Hospital, and then hand-delivered it.

30/12/94

Dad took me to the QE today to see Mr McMaster. He reduced my anti-rejection drugs again. We also saw Dave, who was his usual lovely self. All in all it was a very good visit.

CHAPTER TWELVE

CELEBRATING THE 1000TH LIVER TRANSPLANT

❧

1995

16/01/95

I had a letter from the hospital to say that they can do my operation (stoma reversal) on 7ᵗʰ February. I would like it done the following week, as I don't want to miss Hellen's 21ˢᵗ party.

19/01/95

I made Robert's birthday cake for his party tomorrow. It is a pool table and I am quite pleased with it. I heard from David Mayer's secretary that it is OK for me to have my operation on 14ᵗʰ February.

24/01/95

I went to the dentist this morning to have a scale and polish and to make a further appointment to have antibiotic cover to prevent any infection. I marzipanned Dad's cake later on and made a banner that says 'Graham we can't believe you're 50'. I went to my sign language class after tea.

25/01/95

I did a couple of hours at Boots. When I got home I had some post from Little Aston Hospital about the job I had applied for. I have got an interview next Tuesday. I went to my pottery class later on and made a floppy-sided dish and a teddy bear.

31/01/95

I wore my new pinstripe dress for my interview at Little Aston, and I think it went OK.

02/02/95

Dad's 50th

Dad opened his presents in the evening and I finished icing his cake for his party tomorrow.

03/02/95

Mum and I had our haircut and then I worked at Boots from 12.00 to 2.00 pm. At 7.30pm it was Dad's party. Steve and Russ, the band, were really brilliant. I told Russ that he looked a bit like Freddie Mercury and he took it as a compliment. He dedicated a 'Queen' song to me. How cute! Loads of friends came and we all had a really good time. Uncle Eric was so drunk; he was hilarious with his groovy dancing. I decided to sing with the band for a couple of songs! I haven't had such a good time for ages.

13/02/95

I went into the hospital by train and was examined by a doctor called Justin. He took some blood and was really quite nice. All being well my operation will be tomorrow afternoon.

14/02/95

I was nil by mouth all day and at 3.00 pm Mr Mayer came to say that he couldn't do my operation today, so, hopefully, it will be tomorrow. Ian, from theatre, came to see me and was lovely. Mum and Dad left at about 7.15 pm.

15/02/95

I was a bit anxious today and was nil by mouth from 8.00 am. At 3.00 pm, Ian collected me for theatre. I was back on the ward at 5.30 pm. When I came round, Mr Mayer and the team thought it was funny that I had put a heart-shaped sign on my stoma bag saying 'Happy belated Valentine's Day'.

17/02/95

I had my catheter out and they have stopped my epidural, but I still have the line in my back, which is really itchy. Judy came to see me and Ian came to take me for a walk down the corridor. I have been to the toilet for a poo!! Wow, how amazing.

22/02/95

Mum came in this morning and I went down to the clock tower and had a sandwich with her. Darius came to see me (in his theatre gear!) and said, 'How come one-half of the theatre staff are in love with me?' What a laugh; which half, I want to know. Eric and Emma came in later and brought me a little dog. It's so cute with its tongue hanging out; I really had a good laugh.

24/02/95

Mum collected me and we went home for a lovely rest. Carole came round later on and everyone is amused by my toy dog. I have named him Ian, after the theatre technician.

27/02/95

Mum took me to the QE outpatients to see Mr Buckels. He is so lovely and he took my stitches out. Dave Mootimer asked me if I would speak at the 1000th transplant celebration day, so I have got to write a speech!

28/02/95

I ran in the pancake race today, and would have won if I hadn't dropped the pancake! Alan Williamson, the Mercury photographer, was there and took loads of photos of me, so I will probably be in the paper again next week.

03/03/95

Mum took me to Little Aston Hospital for an interview as Healthcare Assistant. Judy collected me and we went to the Lent lunch together.

07/03/95

I had an early start from Carole's at Harrogate and arrived at Ripon College at 7.30 am. We had several sessions before the main interview, including writing an essay and numerical tests. I really like the college.

08/03/95

I caught the train from Harrogate at 9.15 am and got to Lichfield at 1.10 pm. Mum picked me up and when we got home I had heard from Little Aston, and I have not got the job. I have got another interview at the QE for an auxiliary job.

13/03/95

Not a good day as I heard from Ripon that I have not been given a place on the Project 2000 course. Anyway, I did loads of cooking and have just about sorted my speech for Saturday.

Sally was bitterly disappointed not to be given a place at Ripon, so she decided to phone the college and speak to the interviewer. I listened in to the call and had the greatest difficulty in keeping quiet, as Sally was subjected to a most patronising woman who said that she needed more interview experience. Apparently, in the group session earlier in the day, Sally had corrected the interviewer, who had not heard of the planned national database for registered donors. I think this was a case of 'teacher knows best', and Sally might have been perceived as being a bit cocky even though she was correct! The nursing profession, though, would not be denied for very long!

18/03/95

1000th LIVER TRANSPLANT CELEBRATION

Mum and I went off to Birmingham University where the celebration was being held - it was a wonderful day. Mr McMaster, Dr David Adams and Mr Mayer spoke in the morning, and then there was a photo call of the transplant patients. It was great knowing that all the people walking out of the room had had transplants. We had a lovely lunch and then, in the first session after lunch, I did my talk. It was nerve racking, but I enjoyed it, and loads of people complimented me on it. I am so proud to be a liver transplant patient [number 980!] The evening celebrations were fun, and Dave gave me a lovely hug and kiss. Mr Mayer also gave me a hug, earlier in the day. I bought a T-shirt with 'Liver Unit' on it, and I shall wear it with pride.

21/03/95

It was a lovely day today. I caught the train to the QE for my interview for the auxiliary job. I should hear from them by the weekend.

25/03/95

Mum collected me from the station on the way back from Sheffield and had my post for me. I have got the auxiliary job and I am so pleased.

06/04/95

I had a good morning tidying my cupboard and then wrote a letter to Michael Fabricant [local MP] about prescription charges.

07/04/95

Mum took me to Selly Oak for a medical for my new job, and everything seems OK. I then had an appointment at the liver clinic and saw Dave Mootimer. Next time I'm going to have a test to see if I can be taken off steroids, so I have got the injection for that in my fridge!

24/04/95

It was my first day of training for my new job today. We had lectures on all sorts of things and were also given our uniform, which we have to wear tomorrow.

Seven months post-transplant

03/05/95

I got up at 5.45 am and left the house at 6.15 for my first day on the ward! I followed Diane, another auxiliary, round all day and she is really nice. I am so pleased I am doing this. Well, actually, I can hardly believe that a year ago I was so poorly.

04/05/95

I drove in for my early shift and saw Mr Buckels on the ward. He was quite surprised to see me.

05/05/95

I had an appointment at the liver clinic and saw Dr Elias. He was really pleased for me about the job. He had the results of my latest tests and, as they are normal, I can come off steroids. Excellent, after twelve years!

09/05/95

I was on an early shift again today and one of the patients on our side is very poorly. It's very sad to see, but I shall have to get used to it.

10/05/95

It was nice to have a day off today to do my own thing. I wrote letters to Tina and Lisa, and received a letter from

Michael Fabricant MP saying that I wasn't entitled to free prescriptions.

04/06/95
I went into work early as we were expecting a transplant operation. I asked if I could watch it. It was really interesting. The patient was a sixteen-year-old girl, and it was amazing to see the new kidney fill up with blood and start working.

06/06/95
I was on an early shift again, and held the hand of Sam, the transplant girl, while she had her central line taken out.

30/06/95
When I got home from work, there was a letter from the QE, which I thought was to do with clinic, but it was an appointment for an interview on 11th July, so I am really excited.

11/07/95
I left home at 7.40 am and arrived at the QE at 9.00 am. After a boring talk about Project 2000, I had my interview. They told me straightaway that I had got a place. I was so excited. I went to the liver clinic to tell Julie and then to theatre to tell Ann, who gave me a hug.

26/08/95

We had a very busy shift and I assisted with a biopsy, and helped with the drainage of a cyst. We also had a patient die; it really hit me as I went home. When Mum asked me if I had had a good day, I burst into tears.

04/09/95

I was off work today and spent the morning chasing up accommodation. I finally confirmed that it would be at Heartlands Hospital. In the evening I went with Anthony Hooker, Transplant Co-ordinator, to do a talk on transplants at Tamworth Methodist Church.

This is from her notes for the talk:

I had coped with liver disease since I was 7 years old. I am now nearly 21 and my life is just beginning thanks to my new liver which I had one year ago.

For 8 years I knew that one day I may need a transplant. The disease was controlled with steroids and was such an unpredictable disease no one could ever be very specific and say how long I had got! The liver is such a major organ, when it is diseased it affects a lot of the body's functions.

When I was just 15 the veins in my oesophagus - oesophageal varices — haemorrhaged, so treatment for those was regular gastroscopies to inject the damaged veins. I always knew I had an enlarged spleen so this was in danger of rupturing, which was exactly what it did when I went down a fast moving water chute on holiday at Center Parcs. I had an emergency splenectomy which I recovered from very quickly and thought that was the end of my troubles.

But in March 1991, when I was 19, I was taken ill with unexplained abdominal pain. I was transferred by ambulance from Stafford Hospital to the Queen Elizabeth Hospital in Birmingham. It was discovered that half my small bowel had a blood clot, so yet again I was rushed to theatre for the removal of 171 cm of ileum and the formation of a temporary ileostomy. I was extremely poorly and spent 5 long weeks in hospital.

In the summer I was in and out of hospital for tests. I was extremely jaundiced and knew that soon a transplant would be the option. Sure enough the subject was approached and I was very scared as I had to make the decision if I wanted it - and the choice was mine, not Mum's, not Dad's, but mine. For two weeks only Mum, Dad, and my two brothers knew that I was going to need a transplant. During those two weeks I got used to the idea and knew that it was what I wanted. I went into hospital for the day with my family to see different members of the transplant team to discuss what was going to happen to me.

After 10 weeks of waiting I had the call, which I answered and was so excited. I had a great rush of emotions, laughing and crying and dashing about to get things ready. Within two hours Mum and Dad took me to the QE. I didn't sleep much. I went in to theatre next morning for a 7 hour operation. I don't remember anything of that day. But the day after I remembered all the visitors and being relieved when I came off the ventilator. After 11 days I came out of hospital.

I now know what it is like to have plenty of energy. I now have a waistline instead of needing elasticated skirts because of my swollen and tender tummy.

My Liver Transplant was a gift that I couldn't have managed without and I shall always be eternally grateful to all the dedicated professionals and my wonderful family who have helped to make my life what it is.

I am just about to start my career by training as a nurse in Birmingham.

08/09/95

It was my last shift on East 4B. I took a cake in and it was a good shift. Just before home time they put me in the bath and covered me with shaving foam. They gave me a lovely bouquet of flowers, and I felt quite sad to be leaving.

12/09/95

Mum burnt a candle all day, as it is one year since my liver transplant. I felt really great all day. In the evening I went with Marianne to a nightclub in Tamworth. We had a great dance and I had loads of energy.

So, one year on from her transplant, Sally was looking and feeling fine and about to leave home, to pursue her calling on the Project 2000 nursing course at the University of Central England, Birmingham.

14/09/95

I went into the QE on the train and waited about for a bed so that I could have my biopsy. Eventually, at 5.15 pm, they got round to doing it. The follow up was a bit slack, as a qualified member of staff didn't come to see me until two hours later. I stayed overnight at the hospital.

15/09/95

Mum collected me in the morning and we went off to see my accommodation. It's OK but nothing brilliant, but there we go. Mum gave it a really good clean for me. I am really tired today, as the biopsy has taken it out of me. Andy phoned later on and I had an early night.

17/09/95

Mum and Dad brought me over to my new accommodation and it looks better with all my stuff in it. Later on, I met some of the other students, and seven of us went out for a drink and had a good giggle.

18/09/95

START OF PROJECT 2000 COURSE

I went with Sarah and Penny to college for what was quite a boring day of introductions. I haven't told anyone about having had a liver transplant. All of us students in our accommodation are not very happy as we are paying £35 per week, while at Selly Oak they are only paying £14!

23/09/95

I went into Birmingham this morning and bought a pair of red jeans and a pair of high-heeled shoes. Mum, Dad, and Rob came over in the afternoon. Dad put a shelf up for me and Mum did a dress fitting for my new party dress. We went out for a bite to eat and had a good giggle. When they had gone I watched TV with some of the other students.

Sally had great fun in making up words, and 'bargainacious' was one she used for shopping.

07/10/95
MY 21ST BIRTHDAY

I had my hair cut in the morning and then laid the tables and set the village hall up for the party. I wore my new silk dress that Mum had made. The party was great and Steve and Russ, the band, were on top form. I had rather too much to drink but it was a real good laugh.

10/10/95

I woke up and felt dreadful, so Mum collected me and took me to the doctors. I have got an ear infection, so the doctor gave me some antibiotics.

11/10/95

I slept in till late, and then, later in the afternoon, Mum dropped me off at the station to return to my wonderful little room.

13/10/95

I went to the QE first thing, for a liver clinic appointment. My biopsy results were OK, or as OK as a transplanted liver can be. They took fourteen vials of blood, and I felt quite dizzy later on. Jim, the Scottish nurse who used to live here, came over to see us later on, and we had a good laugh.

15/10/95

I started an embroidery that I'd had for my birthday. After tea, I sat with Karen in the TV room and we had quite an uneventful evening. That was until 10.30 pm, when the fire alarm went off, and we all went outside, while three fire engines arrived. So that brightened up our evening.

17/10/95

We had a great lecture this morning about infection control, by a chap called Carlton Murdoch. He was lovely. We then had Community Studies, which was mega boring. In the evening I spoke to Dad, and then phoned Andy.

18/10/95

We only had a half-day today and had Physiology with Tim Badger. It was very good. I went into town and bought a short-patterned black skirt and a black jumper, both for a bargain £8.49!

24/10/95

An OK day at college, and then I phoned Auntie Barbara, as I was dying to know how Clare was. She had a baby boy at 11.55 am, and he is almost 8lb.

25/10/95

We had a half-day at college, and then I went into town to get something for Clare's baby boy, James. I bought a pair of dungarees and two pairs of mega tiny socks. I went over to see Clare and her baby, James Alfred, he is so beautiful. I had a lovely cuddle.

07/11/95

Mum rang me this morning, to say that James Harle had been taken into Birmingham Children's Hospital with a heart problem. I was worried all morning, so I went over to see him after surgery. It was awful to see him with drips, drains, and a ventilator.

10/11/95

I went to see James first thing, and he had just been moved out of ICU. He looked beautiful but still a bit yellow.

Sally ended the year settled in her new accommodation, really enjoying the nursing course, and making lots of new friends. It was always a joy to welcome her back on her frequent trips 'home'.

CHAPTER THIRTEEN

HARD NOT TO CRY

1996

03/01/96

All afternoon and evening, I continued with my Mr Men drawings. I have done A5 pictures of different Mr Men for all my friend's doors! What a laugh!

04/01/96

I packed up all my stuff, ready to return to Gloucester House tomorrow. I slept in Robert's room again, so we were giggling for ages before we went to sleep.

19/01/96

I was at the QE first thing, for a liver clinic appointment. Hopefully, they are going to tidy up my scar soon. After college, I zoomed off home on the train, and Dad picked me up.

08/03/96

I went to college first thing and then to liver clinic. I saw Mr Mayer and he was lovely as usual. He is going to refer me to a plastic surgeon about my scar. Later on I caught the train home and Dad picked me up.

24/04/96

Mum's Birthday

When Mum came back from work, I packed all my stuff and we went back to Birmingham. I had an appointment at Selly Oak Hospital with Mr Peart, a plastic surgeon. He was great, so I am going to have something done about my messy scars.

18/05/96

I went over to Mum and Dad's and my project for the weekend is to make a bright yellow satin blouse. Later on, Mum and Dad went to the cinema, and Rob and I had a laugh watching the Eurovision Song Contest; it was a load of rubbish.

03/07/96

Mum picked me up at 3.00 pm and took me to the Selly Oak Burns and Plastic Surgery Unit. I had a blood test and my tummy drain inserted. The girl in the next bed is having a breast reduction.

04/07/96

The anaesthetist came to see me first thing and I went down to theatre at about 1.15 pm. Mum was waiting for me when I came back. I have had a morphine infusion, so I am feeling dead dopey.

Mum and Andy came to see me and, later on, Dad and Rob. Mr Peart took my dressings off to look at my flat tummy and a very neat scar!

06/07/96

I had my drain out this morning, and then, after lunch, Dad collected me and took me home.

15/07/96

I went to the Liver Support Group meeting in the evening, and was elected as the publicity person, so that should be a laugh.

Sally proved to be very active in promoting the Liver Support Group and would later on use her publicity skills in promoting the cause of transplantation.

24/07/96

I went into college and had it confirmed that I can progress to stage two, but Karen, Elaine, and Liam are off the course. When we got back, Karen was really upset.

18/09/96

I was in theatre again today with Dave. We had a busy day, and had to calm two children who were going to theatre. There was a bit more blood around today, as the surgeon hit an artery; what a flyer that was!

19/09/96

I was on the maternity unit today. They did a Caesarean section and I watched it all. The mum had a little girl and it was a magical experience. It was hard not to cry.

04/11/96

I was on an early shift, which was a bit messy. Afterwards I went for a smear test and picked up my prescription. I feel really tearful tonight. It didn't help seeing a letter in my notes file from Dr Elias to my GP. It was on 13/08/94 and said 'Sally's bilirubin★ level is 544 and so has not got long left'.

★Bilirubin is a natural substance produced by the liver, but an unusually high level indicates that all is not well.

06/11/96

I was in theatre to watch an operation. It was interesting to see the lungs, and I could see the heart pumping. After work I had a little doze and then went to a Liver Support Group meeting.

13/11/96

I had a phone call from one of the nurses to tell me that the overdose patient, who was in the next bed to me after my transplant and who subsequently recovered, had committed suicide. I am so upset; it's awful.

As part of the Project 2000 course, Sally would have many varied placements in hospitals, health centres, care homes, and schools.

15/11/96

I really enjoyed my school placement today. We had an aromatherapy session, massaging the children's hands and feet. Later on they had their celebrations for Divali, which was fun. I phoned Emma and am going to see her in Nottingham on Sunday.

18/11/96

I was in a different class at school today, and they were so naughty. One of the children bit me! After tea I went to a Liver Patient's Support meeting.

19/11/96

I went into school today in the snow, and the children were a bit better behaved. However, one of the girls kicked me in the mouth, so I have got a thick lip.

21/11/96

I met Beverley Cornforth at the QE and we went to Alcester Grammar School to give a talk on transplants. I was quite proud of myself answering some of the questions that the children asked.

23/11/96

I met Dad in Lichfield at the Peugeot garage, and test-drove a 306, which I am having next week. I can't wait as nobody else knows about it.

24/11/96

I met Emma at Aston University and we both went over to Nottingham to see Sue. It was absolutely lovely meeting up with them both. There had been a weather warning about snow, so we set off back after lunch.

29/11/96

I had a good last day at school, and they gave me a card and a mug filled with sweets. Later on, I met Andy in Lichfield and we did a spot of shopping. I received some exciting news, that in the New Year, I am going to be on Sky TV with John Buckels and Beverley Cornforth, promoting organ donation!

31/12/96

I was up early helping Mum prepare for the party. It was a snowy day and very cold. We had a fun party with lots of silly games and a bit of wild dancing at midnight.

CHAPTER FOURTEEN

LETTERS TO GRANDMA AND GRANDDAD

❧

1997

Sally continued to write her diary but, unfortunately, the entries for several years have been lost. However, we do have some of the letters that Sally wrote to her grandparents. Writing letters, postcards and little messages was something that Sally was very good at. Mr Men characters and little smiley faces often made an appearance on the letters.

Sally was continuing her nursing training, which included several placements on wards in different hospitals. These placements, along with the mentoring she received, gave Sally a tremendous grounding and confidence in all aspects of nursing. The experiences included contact with patients and relatives, assisting doctors with medical procedures, taking patients to theatre, attending surgical operations, installing and removing catheters, looking after bays of patients and handing over after night shifts, admitting patients and administering drugs and blood and saline drips. She was also promoting the cause of transplantation, appearing in 'The Nursing Times' and other publications, television interviews as well as giving presentations to schools etc. After one of her hospital placements Sally writes, *This was a fantastic placement which has filled me with confidence. I would like very much like to work in ITU in the future.*

Sally was also making new friends, including a new boyfriend, Mike Painting, in May 1997. Here are some extracts from those letters:

Tuesday 17th June 1997
Dear Grandma and Granddad,
I did buy some postcards, but not enough, so I thought I'd send you some of my groovy Mr Men paper! Scotland is as beautiful as ever and Angela, Mum and I have had a lovely walk around the coast. We all went to St. Andrews yesterday. It is such a lovely place, but a bit too much golf for us lasses. Angela and I have been swimming every morning before breakfast. The week beginning 30th June is National Transplant week and I am going to be featured in The Nursing Times. I've got three assignments due in the same week at college, as well as a test, so I shall be really rather busy.
Lots of sunny smiles, hugs and kisses from Scotland
Love Sally.

Angela became a close friend, having met Sally in the nursing home at Heartlands.

Monday 30th June 1997
Dear Grandma and Granddad,
Thanks for your letter and it was lovely to speak to Granddad on Saturday. I'm glad the new gluten-free diet is going OK. I did another talk with Beverley [transplant co-ordinator] *to students at a school in Bourneville and it went very well. National Transplant Week started with a service in Birmingham Cathedral, which was extremely emotional. I burst into tears as I was finishing my speech. The service was entitled 'The Precious Gift'. Whilst I was waiting for my transplant, the idea of someone else's liver inside me bothered me from time to time. It upset me that in order for my life to be maintained, someone else had to die. One of the first things I wanted to do after my transplant was to express my gratitude to my donor family. It was the hardest letter I have ever written, but I felt extremely at peace after I had sent it. I have never felt guilty about being alive due to someone else's misfortune, as I know the organ was donated to me as a gift, and it is that precious gift of life I shall always treasure.*

Mum and I are looking forward to going on the train to London on Wednesday to promote the donor card.

I don't know if Mum has told you, but I have a new boyfriend, and I have been seeing him for two months. His name is Mike and he is taking me out for a meal tonight, so I had better look through my wardrobe for something nice to wear.

Sally and her mum had a great day out in London promoting the transplant donor card. They travelled down on the train, handing out donor cards on the way. They then made their way to Wimbledon and spent a very pleasant afternoon watching the tennis, before travelling home handing out more cards. They bought a copy of 'Nursing Times' on Euston Station. Sally was on the front page!

Wednesday 24th September1997
Dear Grandma and Granddad,
…I've just had a Hepatitis B injection, and it hurt! I've got a day off college, so I am catching up on washing and ironing. So what did you think of Mike? Tall!
P.S. Hope the sausages were OK.

Monday 27th October 1997
…I started my placement last Monday in the Intensive Care Department at the Queen Elizabeth Hospital. It's great but it is a bit weird as it brings back so many memories.

Friday 12th December 1997

….It was lovely to see you on Wednesday and spend some time with you both. I had a very energetic time at Line Dancing, and didn't get back till late. I start a new placement next week, and after that I only have two more before I qualify.

CHAPTER FIFTEEN

GRADUATION AND A GOLD MEDAL

❦

1998

This was the year when Sally would fulfil her calling and qualify as a nurse.

Tuesday 13th January 1998
Dear Grandma and Granddad,
…I am busy preparing for tomorrow, as I am doing a teaching session with some of the staff on hand massage. That should be nice and relaxing and something a bit different. Mike and I are going to the hospital ball next week. Mike bought himself a dinner suit last weekend and I got him a dress shirt and bow tie for Christmas, so he should look a bit of a smarty pants! Only eight months left until I qualify.

Sally continued her training, including various placements and the next letter to her grandparents shows her excitement as she approached qualification and also her enjoyment of 'hands on' experience!

Saturday 8th August 1998
Dear Grandma and Granddad,
…I've got just two more weeks on placement plus a week in college before I finish. I had my last two assignments back last week and I passed them both. I've now received my new uniforms all ready for being a staff nurse! On Thursday I went into theatre for the day to watch some bowel surgery. It was great. I scrubbed up so I could assist the surgeon. I held a retractor out of the way and had the patient's bowel in my hand to make it easier for the surgeon to see inside. So, I had my hands inside the patient's abdomen. It was great!!

It is my Graduation Ball on the 21st August and my posh frock is all finished.
Lots of love, hugs, and sunshine smiles
Sally
Xxxx

On 21st September 1998 Sally started work as a staff nurse at Heartlands Hospital, Birmingham. She had achieved her dream and vocation by being the first person to train and qualify as a nurse after receiving a life-saving liver transplant. Could anyone be better qualified for the nursing profession?

Sally's grandma had to move into a nursing home in Tamworth in December and Sally continued to visit her there whenever she could.

Sally's graduation took place at the Symphony Hall, Birmingham on the 5th February 1999. It would be difficult to say who was the proudest on this wonderful day; Sally, Michael or her doting parents. The following is an entry in the visitors book at the nursing home where Sally's Grandma was resident.

Thursday 11th March 1999
I arrived to see Grandma at 9.30 am. Grandma was in the dining room and was just finishing off her cup of tea with breakfast. Her face lit up when she saw me. One of the carers helped Grandma back to her room. Then another carer (I don't know her name but she often sings to her - she's a lovely lady) brought us a tray of coffee and biscuits. I helped Grandma drink her coffee as she is finding it difficult to hold her cup. Grandma really did enjoy her one and a half cups! It's now 10.45 am and I shall soon be off to see dad. Love to whoever writes in here next. Sally xx

Later that day, Sally's grandma was rushed from the nursing home to hospital but, sadly, passed away on route. Sally was the last close relative to see her before she died.

Sally had always enjoyed swimming, so she grabbed the opportunity to take part in the British Transplant games, to be held in Birmingham in June. She trained diligently for it and even had a session with an Olympic swimmer, Nick Gillingham, who had come along to a training session as part of the publicity for the games. In the event, he spent some time with Sally, helping her to perfect her tumble turns.

After competing and winning a couple of medals she was invited to take part in the World Transplant Games which would be held in Budapest in the following September. This involved a degree of sponsorship which we managed to arrange very quickly. Along with her boyfriend Mike, we duly booked our flights for this exciting venture. We were all to discover just how competitive transplant patients could be.

We eventually arrived in Budapest and booked into the hotel which had been arranged for us. The hotel was adequate - apart from the food and service! After experiencing a couple of evening meals we all decided to go in to town to seek better food. On the first occasion our taxi was involved in a minor accident and we transferred to another taxi while the combatants sorted out liability. Thankfully, the meal was worth the effort.

The welcome ceremony for all the competitors and supporters was held in Heroes Square, where all the different nationalities gathered in groups and we listened to speeches and enjoyed the band and outside dancing.

Sally, not being a natural competitor, was extremely nervous before each race but, despite the nerves, won first bronze, then silver and finally, in the four-leg relay, a gold. We were privileged to attend a reception at the British Embassy and the week-long activities culminated in a wonderful gala dinner and firework display.

At the closing ceremony, in the national arena, it was wonderful to see so many transplant patients gathered together in one place.

In November Sally and I went along to the Civic Hall, Lichfield for the annual Darwin Lecture organised by the Lichfield Science and Engineering Society. The lecture was given by Professor Paul McMaster, who was the joint founder of the Transplant Unit at Queen Elizabeth Hospital, Birmingham. His subject was 'Transplant Surgery in the Next Millennium'. After he had delivered his address, I stood up to ask a question, or rather to thank him for giving me my daughter back. On seeing Sally sitting beside me he invited her down onto the stage, saying that she could deliver a far better lecture than he could!

CHAPTER SIXTEEN

PROUD FATHER OF THE BRIDE

✤

2000

In January, while they were walking on the Tissington Trail, Mike asked Sally to marry him and, of course, she said yes. They then drove to our house, where Sally concealed the ring from Val while Mike did the traditional thing of asking me for her hand in marriage. I also said yes!

We were all over the moon and it soon became clear that they were intent on getting married that year. We set about finding a venue for the reception and booked Longdon Church for the ceremony. The date was set for the 16th September, which just happened to be my mum's birthday.

Sally and Mike set about house hunting and finally found one in Great Barr. Val and I had a pre-wedding holiday and on our return, Sally and Mike picked us up from the airport and drove us to their new house.

Val is a trained dressmaker and therefore it was inevitable that she would make Sally's wedding dress. Oh, and five bridesmaid dresses as well! The theme for the bridesmaid dresses? Rainbow colours of course!

Walking Sally into church was without doubt the proudest moment of my life. The Rev John Allen married them and both Rev Robert Ellis and Rev Peter Holliday took part in the service. Andy was chief usher and Rob drove my car to ferry Val and one of the bridesmaids. A friend supplied a beautiful American Case motor car for the bride, father of the bride and the other four bridesmaids to church, and for the newly-weds to the reception. We all had a wonderful day.

As if preparing for the wedding was not enough to do, Sally spotted an advertisement for a vacancy at the Queen Elizabeth Hospital and duly applied. There was never any doubt that she would get the job, so she was now working on the very ward where she had been a patient. Sally was welcomed with open arms by nurses, doctors and surgeons alike. Very soon the doctors were simply 'her boys', a title they accepted with good grace from this cheeky new recruit!

During this year Andy met Rachel and it was great that she was able to come to the wedding and meet all the family. Sally and Rachel soon became great friends.

2001

One of the highlights of 2001 for me was shopping with Sally. Not just any old shop, but helping me to choose a dress for Val, which I had never had the confidence to buy. We decided that Lichfield had enough dress shops so surely, we could find something suitable. Sally had the ability to turn any activity into a fun experience.

After trying on several dresses in several different shops, we ventured into a fairly 'posh' shop with what proved to be a fairly 'pushy' assistant. After trying on several garments Sally eventually chose a particularly classy and expensive dress to try on. To try to clinch the sale the assistant asked Sally what her 'partner' thought of it. This was the first time I had been mistaken for a sugar daddy and, of course, Sally thought it was hilarious. We made a fairly quick exit from the shop before we were both overcome with fits of the giggles.

We eventually chose and purchased a dress. Unfortunately, it wasn't to Val's liking, so she took it back and exchanged it, but I wouldn't have missed the experience for the world.

2002

Every year the International Transplant Nurses' Society holds a symposium, usually in America. For 2002 it would be held in Pittsburgh. Sally was offered a place on the trip and didn't need to be asked twice, so, along with colleagues Moira, Tracey and Helen, they set off. When they got there Sally and Helen were so giggly and excited at the luxury of the hotel rooms that Moira had to apologise to the bell boy!

One of the keynote speakers at the seminar was Professor Thomas Starzl, the pioneer of liver transplantation in America. After his speech they heard someone at the microphone. It was Sally. She said 'Professor Starzl, you don't know me but my name is Sally and I had a transplant under Professor Paul Mc Master in Birmingham' [this information had not been imparted to any of the girls that Sally had met at the symposium, until that moment] 'and I just wanted to say thank you for all you have done, because without you I wouldn't be here today'. It blew everyone away!

Apart from attending the talks, they spent a day on the Liver Ward in the Pittsburgh Hospital, where they were made very welcome. They also went swimming in the hotel pool, did some serious dress shopping, went to a baseball game, and attended a gala dinner on a riverboat, where they met one of Professor Starzl's theatre nurses, who were singing with the jazz band. A pretty full trip then!

2003

January 18th was Rob's 21st birthday and the highlight of the party was Rob making his entrance in a huge teddy bear's costume to the sound of 'Let me entertain you'. Not content with entertaining everyone at the party, he donned the outfit again at a family get-together at home the next day and proceeded to walk around the village, much to the consternation of passing motorists, police and pedestrians!

Sally was working long shifts as a newly-promoted sister at the Queen Elizabeth Hospital and Mike continued to work nearby as an engineering draughtsman. They enjoyed entertaining in their home, as well as setting about decorating and improving the house. We enjoyed the fact that they lived nearby for all the special visits.

Meanwhile, Andy had proposed to Rachel and began their preparations for their big day. Sally was to be a bridesmaid along with Ruth, Rachel's sister.

In September, the co-founder of the transplant unit at the Queen Elizabeth Hospital, Professor Paul

McMaster, retired. Sally asked to speak at the gala evening held in his honour. According to consultant surgeon Darius Mirza, despite Paul's request to keep the evening low key, Sally spoke beautifully and eloquently, and reduced everyone to tears of joy.

2004

This year had all the potential to be very special. Andrew and Rachel were busy planning their wedding and we were delighted that they had suggested it be held at our house. We did what we could to extend the lawn to provide maximum space for the marquee.

Val and I decided to treat ourselves to a pre-wedding Caribbean cruise. We dropped heavy hints to Sally and Mike and eventually, they decided to come with us. On the 12th March we flew off to Barbados to begin our ten-day holiday. We all had the most marvellous time visiting beautiful islands and Sally certainly enjoyed dressing up for dinner in some of the dresses she had bought in Pittsburgh. I know I am a bit biased, but she looked absolutely stunning.

It was a good job we had a special and relaxing time, because a few weeks after we got back we had a flash flood which caused havoc in the garden as well as ruining carpets in the house. Our first thought was to wonder what we were going to do with only five weeks to the wedding, but with a lot of hard work and the co-operation of decorators, carpet fitters and other tradesmen, we recovered by the 29th May. The rain finally stopped in the morning, and glorious sunshine blessed this special day.

We had another very special day on August 15th, our wedding anniversary. Sally and Mike came to see us to tell us the news that Sally was expecting a baby. Needless to say, we were over the moon. Rob was thrilled at the thought of becoming an uncle.

Val decided to write a diary addressed to the precious baby Sally was carrying, extracts of which appear in Chapter 18. Val imagined our first grandchild reading this some time in the future, and so she recorded her innermost thoughts as well as the significant events as the pregnancy progressed.

Ten days after sharing the news with us, Sally and Mike joined us for a few days on holiday in Wales. We enjoyed walking, chatting, and swimming as we all enjoyed the sea air in Aberdovey. September 3rd was Sally's first scan, confirming everything was healthy and adding a touch of reality to the situation.

September 12th was the tenth anniversary of Sally's transplant and plans were well in hand for the triple celebration of that, her 30th birthday and going public on the secret that the close family was still keeping.

September 29th saw the publication of the hospital's in-house magazine, 'Patient Focus', with Sally's glorious smile beaming out on the front cover. The article inside detailed Sally's amazing journey from transplant to working on the very same ward that gifted her new life.

October 7th was Sally's birthday and, two days later, the most wonderful party with family and friends. David Mayer, Sally's transplant surgeon and one of her 'Boys' was there with his wife and was overjoyed to propose the toast , after revealing the news of her pregnancy.

Val's dad, who was looking forward to becoming a resident of Longdon, enjoyed the celebrations along with everyone else.

Over the coming weeks Val and Sally spent lots of time together whether shopping for the baby, knitting, hospital visits for scans and check-ups, or just simply chatting. They were also very much involved in planning for my forthcoming 60th birthday party.

CHAPTER SEVENTEEN

NO, NO, PLEASE NO!

2005

On January 25th 2005, Sally woke up in acute pain and Mike rushed through the morning traffic to the Birmingham Women's Hospital, where she underwent an emergency caesarean operation. Sadly, the baby, though perfect at 29 weeks, was born in distress and did not survive resuscitation.

Mike telephoned me at my office to say that Sally had lost the baby and was asking for us. I dashed home without saying a word to anyone and tried to contact Val at a friend's house. I knew that Val had planned to go swimming with her friend, Shirley, so I left a message at the leisure centre, asking them to tell Val to meet me at home as soon as possible.

When Val arrived home, she burst into tears on hearing the news, but had guessed that something was wrong. Rob then arrived home, after the office staff had told him of my abrupt departure. In my turmoil I had not even thought to tell him the awful news.

All three of us then set off to the hospital. When we arrived and saw the baby in a cot in the recovery room, Sally said 'This is your grandson, Edward Graham, and he is perfect'. I burst into tears and Sally asked Mike to comfort me. Sally always put other people first.

She asked each one of us to kiss her, and throughout the day she kept telling Mike how much she loved him. Was she aware of something seriously wrong inside her?

I telephoned Andy, and his wife, Rachel, who were living and working in London, and they immediately set off to join us. A little later on, Mike's parents, George and Barbara, also joined us. We all held the baby, each one of us lost in our own thoughts of what might have been, and what so nearly was. Our good friend Peter Holliday came in the afternoon, and spent some time with us.

Sally was being constantly monitored by the doctors, and it became obvious that all was not well. The doctors considered transferring her to the Queen Elizabeth Hospital nearby, but decided that it was too risky to move her. She continued to deteriorate, and at 6.30 pm she was rushed to theatre. Andy and Rachel arrived shortly afterwards.

Shortly after 9 pm, the senior surgeon, Darius Mirza, came to see us, and it was clear from his demeanour that something terrible had happened. He led us to a private room and I will remember that short walk for the rest of my life. I kept repeating 'No, no, please no!' to myself, but the awful news was broken to us that Sally had died on the operating table, despite their best efforts to save her.

I somehow managed to keep myself together to question and thank the surgeon, while the rest of the family were sobbing in total shock. This was our worst nightmare. Sally had been in serious trouble many times before, but had always recovered; not this time.

Mike's brother, Stephen, arrived, and I telephoned and left a message for Peter Holliday, who arrived around midnight. We all gathered around Sally's bed, not wanting to believe what had happened, but our eyes could not deny it. Mike decided to stay at Sally's bedside for the remainder of the night and Stephen agreed to stay with him. The rest of us went home to try to sleep.

We awoke next morning to the awful realisation that we had not had a bad dream; the events of the previous day were all too real. One of the first things we had to do was to tell Len, Sally's Granddad, who had moved to Longdon only weeks before, to be closer to us.

The only thing we could now do for Sally was to arrange her funeral. Before that could happen, a post mortem had to be carried out because of the suddenness of her death. Mike made the necessary arrangements, for which I was grateful, as it was something I had to totally blank out of my mind.

We went over to Mike's house to meet with the undertaker, who agreed with our request to have the funeral on Saturday 5th February, despite the fact that they did not usually carry out funerals on a Saturday. We also agreed to ask Peter Holliday and John Allen to take part in the funeral service, which would take place in St James in Longdon. John Allen had married Sally and Mike there just over four years before.

Rob set about compiling two CDs of Sally's favourite music; one to be played prior to the funeral service, and the other at the village hall afterwards.

We set aside time every day to open and read the hundreds of cards and letters which the postman delivered. It was clear that Sally had touched the lives of very many people.

On the day before the funeral, we were collecting flowers from a florist in Lichfield when we heard live music being played across the street. The song was 'Somewhere over the Rainbow'; just another of those coincidences.

The day of the funeral inevitably arrived. The weather was cold but with bright sunshine as the funeral cortege made its way from Sally and Mike's house in Great Barr to Longdon Church. The church was packed; it was standing room only. Tributes were given by Sally's consultant, Professor Elwyn Elias, and by Annie Jones, a dear friend and our yoga tutor, who challenged each of the congregation to focus on just one of Sally's many gifts.

Sally's friend and colleague Helen Hewitt delivered a reading entitled 'Laughter', which Sally had copied out and framed ten years before. Cousin David had composed a musical tribute entitled 'Sketches for Sally and Edward', which he movingly played on the piano.

Peter Holliday read out reflections written by Val and Andy, and John Allen did the same for Mike and Rob. Peter also gave the main address. I somehow managed to deliver my own thoughts, with Annie standing beside me for much-needed support. We left the church to the strains of 'Love Changes Everything'.

Later on it poured with rain. One of Rob's chosen songs was 'Tears in Heaven'.

★ ★ ★

It was not until after the funeral that the true awfulness of what had happened sank in. A light had been switched off permanently, and we were left wondering how we could possibly cope without Sally.

The staff at the hospital, Sally's friends and colleagues, suggested that we should hold a memorial service, and we were fortunate to be able to hold this in St Philip's Cathedral in Birmingham. The service was arranged and led by the hospital's chaplain, Francis Buxton. There were musical contributions from organist Matt Penn, violinist Peter Hartley, pianist David Jenkinson. A CD was played of the song 'Sally Sunshine', and there was a very special rendition of 'You are my sunshine' by the hospital staff music group.

There were readings and tributes by colleagues Moira Perrin, David Mayer, and Graham Lipkin and our friend Robert Ellis. Rob and Andy read moving tributes. Rob read words he had written entitled 'Dear Sally' and Andy read a poem I had written. Both of these can be found in the appendix.

On Sally's birthday, when she would have been 31, we arranged a fund-raising dance for friends and colleagues at Drayton Manor where Rob and his friends Richard, Peter, Matt and Sarah provided the live music.

We had already opened a bank account in the name of 'The Sally Painting Memorial Fund' and would later formalise this into a charitable trust. We decided to focus support on the Liver Unit at The Queen Elizabeth Hospital. This took the form of supporting therapeutic treatments for liver patients both pre and post-transplant. We never intended to throw ourselves into fundraising, although several relatives and friends held various sponsored events. These included nurse Rachel Howells running in the 2006 London Marathon, Rob doing a skydive in Australia, a golf day organised by my brother, Eric, and a group of doctors and nurses entering the Great North Run half marathon under the name of 'Team Sally'. The most touching of all was a climb of Mount Kilimanjaro where Sally's friend and colleague, Helen Hewitt, placed a pebble on the summit which her children had painted with Sally's initials and a rainbow. We hoped the charity would be a receptacle for donations from family and friends of patients in receipt of life-saving transplants at the Queen Elizabeth Hospital, Birmingham.

CHAPTER EIGHTEEN

EDWARD'S DIARY

❧

When Sally and Mike told us they were expecting a baby, our first grandchild, we were totally overjoyed. Val decided to keep a diary for baby Painting dedicated to 'Granvie's Little Treasure' Granvie is not a miss-spelling of 'grannie' - it is what Val had decided she would like be known as.

DEDICATED TO GRANVIE'S LITTLE TREASURE

Monday August 16th 2004
A beautiful candle lit for a little one. I wonder what colour it is.
The candle is a beautiful shade of purple.
My heart is bursting with warmth.

Wednesday August 17th
Mummy is radiant! I met her to try on posh frocks.
You are at the energy level of Svadistana – the glow of orange, the second colour of the rainbow. A ray of light.

Thursday August 19th

Today I walked about 8 miles on Cannock Chase with your great-granddad. He doesn't know about you yet. I know I am very special to him and you will be just as special to your dad. My dad was so excited when he knew your mum was on the way. I can't wait for her to tell him about you.

My dad is 87 years old. When you are born he will be 88! I have lit a candle every day since I knew you were on the way.

Friday August 20th

Today we looked at the Passey family tree. You will be the start of the next generation, even though you will be a little Painting. It was a miserable rainy day, but I never noticed. I'm full of sunshine inside – because of you.

Today's candle is orange, like a jewel, floating in a glass of water.

Saturday August 21st

Instead of lighting a candle, we thought of you at the seaside. We walked along the beach from Aberdovey to Towyn , looking at the pebbles. I tried to find one about your size.

Sunday August 22nd

We lit candles for you in Pennal church. Most of the congregation were Welsh and some of the service was spoken in Welsh. Not the sermon though, which was about things growing from something small and making a difference. Never underestimate the difference you can make. You are tiny, tiny and already you have made a difference to my life.

Monday August 23rd
Today is Alex's 21st birthday. He is your second cousin, and doesn't know about you yet.

We lit the World Peace Flame today. Let's hope the world will become a more peaceful place in your lifetime.

Thursday August 26th
Your mum and dad came to stay with us at Plas Talgarth. Your mum has always loved jelly babies and she brought some with her. We thought that you were not as big as a jelly baby yet!

Friday August 27th
We all had a long walk along the beach at Aberdovey. We talked a lot about how exciting it will be to share the news of you with all the family. You had your first swim!

Friday September 3rd
Today was your first scan. I was looking forward all morning to the telephone call to say that all was well. The scan confirmed your size; only 15mm! Wow, so tiny!

Sunday September 5th

We saw your scan photo today and we are all so excited.

I lit a candle in St James Church. During the service we were all given a Malteser, and I had a lovely thought that you would be small enough to fit inside one!

We met with Paul and Pauline (Andy's in-laws) for tea and a major planning session for your mum's 30th birthday party. It's going to be a great do.

Saturday September 11th

All week I have been waiting for today because your mum and dad are telling your Uncle Andrew and Auntie Rachel about you. Andrew rang us so excited about the news.

Sunday September 12th

It is 10 years since your mum's transplant and, because of that you will be even more special to everyone.

It is the Longdon Produce Show and I was delighted to win first prize for my floral art entry entitled 'The children's party'. I so enjoyed doing it! Lots of people congratulated me, but they didn't know that I was inspired by you and all the parties we will enjoy with you in the future!

Saturday September 18th

Today I walked 10 miles on the Staffordshire Way with my WI friends. Several of them asked after your mum. They usually say 'how is your daughter?' If they say that next month I will be able to tell them about you!

After I got home, your great-granddad came along with Andy and Rachel and your mum and dad. We were all together when great-granddad heard the news. They told him it was still top secret. It's exciting keeping a secret, but I can't wait for everyone to know!

Wednesday September 29th
Today there is an amazing article in a magazine about your mum working on the Liver Unit. I read it over and over again. Your mum is like a beacon, giving out loads of light and joy to all around her; and you have given her even more radiance.

The article was in 'Patient Focus', the Queen Elizabeth Hospital magazine.

Thursday September 30th
Today I discovered a tiny oak tree which must have grown from an acorn dropped by a squirrel. It was 22cm high. It was in a perfect spot, so we dedicated the tree to you. I expect you will overtake it in height at some stage; it should grow taller than all of us.

Thursday October 7th
Today is your mum's birthday and she came over and had lunch with me. We were planning the special party and talking about you a lot.

Friday October 8ᵗʰ

Your second scan. It is so marvellous that it shows you are 12 weeks plus 2 days.

Saturday October 9ᵗʰ

We had the most wonderful party for your mum with the great announcement to all the friends about you. I wondered about the loudness of the music affecting you. We sang a great rendition of 'You make me wanna shout'! There was so much joy and fun.

Thursday October 15ᵗʰ

I am planning a yoga session for next week at Streetly, where your mum attends a class. You have inspired me in what I am going to do. The music I will use is 'If I only had you, I could change the world'.

Sunday October 17ᵗʰ

Today I planted some daffodil bulbs in the garden. I thought of you and whether they might be just out when you are born. I think I will plan a rainbow of flowers for next year.

Saturday October 30ᵗʰ

I have been to Egypt with your great granddad to see the place he served in during the war. We enjoyed meeting with veterans and their families.

Today we had tea at your mum and dad's house. Your mum looks absolutely radiant. She has gone up a dress size but you are still only 11 cm long. Your heart beat has been heard and you have fingernails already!

Sunday November 21st
We watched a programme on television about your mum's work on the Liver Unit, and the patients who receive donor organs. I thought you probably were on this ward at that moment as your mum was on duty.

Tuesday November 23rd
I heard your heartbeat today! I went along with your mum to the clinic. I could hear lots of swishy noises; then a perfect thud, thud, thud.

Thursday November 25th
We are a step nearer moving Great Granddad to Longdon. The bungalow is looking bare as it is being cleared.

Friday December 10th
We heard that you were in hospital. I expect it is because you are active and letting us know your presence. We are thinking of you constantly, and praying for your safety. Xx

Saturday December 18th

Today I lit a candle for you in Great Granddad's new bungalow. We have had a busy two days preparing for him to move to Longdon. He felt you kicking today.

Saturday December 25th

There are a lot of lovely things going on but, unfortunately, your mum and dad had to go to the hospital as your mum was not feeling very well. We all had a very late night waiting for news, but the best thing was hearing your heartbeat. Your granddad was very excited.

Sunday December 26th

There has been a disaster in the Far East; a huge tidal wave. We are thinking a lot of Uncle Andrew and Auntie Rachel as they have gone to Thailand on holiday.

Monday December 27th

You have been observed on the scan again and your little toes can be seen. It is Great Uncle Peter's 60th birthday today. We had a lovely walk with them and their friends.

Thursday December 30th

I have been writing the special invitations for your granddad's 60th birthday in February. One of the features of the party will be 'Granddad's Resolutions'. There are 60 of them and you occupy quite a few. Guests are being asked to bring an item which will help him achieve the resolutions.

Friday December 31ˢᵗ

I was 'Cinderella' at a New Year's Eve Party. We saw the New Year in at Stoneyfield's farm , and the first thing I thought was I AM GOING TO BE A GRANDMUM THIS YEAR!

Monday January 3ʳᵈ

Today your great granddad moved into Longdon. Your mum, dad, Robert, and Great Uncle Peter all helped. By the end of the day he was well settled in.

Sunday January 9ᵗʰ

Your granddad, Robert, Richard, Sarah, and Matt all rehearsed for the birthday party songs.

Friday January 14ᵗʰ

I took your mum in for her next scan, and was able to stay and watch. I was so excited! First we heard all the swishy sounds, and then we could see your shapes appearing on the screen, all moving about. We soon made out a clear picture of your little foot and then your feet and hands. We could see your spine and all the vertebrae, your head, your cute little *nose and lips. We then saw you yawn and put your tongue out! Your weight is approximately 2lb 7ozs.*

Tuesday January 18th
Today is Uncle Robert's 23rd Birthday. I am reminded that he was the last family member to be born. I think he will be very glad that I will stop calling him 'my baby' as you will adopt that title soon!

Friday January 21st
Your mum is in hospital again, but this time she is content that all is well. You are now 28 weeks and 2 days old. Judging by the amount of movement you create you must be fit.

Granddad's log cabin is on the way and he has some lovely plans for using it, and I am sure you will have a special time there.

The diary abruptly ends there. The cabin duly arrives on January 25th, the day I get the dreadful telephone call from Mike to say that Sally had lost the baby. Edward would never get to read the heartfelt words from Granvie.

FINAL REFLECTIONS

So how do you cope? How do you find meaning in life's tragedies? How do you express the inexpressible? How do you recover from having your faith tested to the limit? I don't have the answers; just the questions.

But what would Sally have made of the outpouring of grief and the desire by so many people to 'do' something in her memory? What is perfectly clear is the way she touched so many lives for the better.

Well there it is. My beautiful daughter, who was responsible for the happiest, proudest, and saddest days of my life, is no longer with us.

Back in 1987 Sally had written in her precious diary; 'perhaps, maybe, someone will publish my diaries'.

Someone just did.

'DEAR SALLY'
by Robert Passey

This comes from the heart
I know no other way
It's your little bro here
Mr Bobs you might say
I hear your voice
All the time in my head
If you were here now
LET'S PARTY you would have said
Thank you for your laughter
And those silly jokes we made
The memories are priceless
They will never fade
So when we think of you
It's always Sal, with that big smile
And a laugh that was like no other
I could hear it from over a mile
That dark night in January
Is forever on my mind
When you were taken from us
You left so much love behind
That love is still so strong
And it's inside everyone here today
I wish you were back with us

To take this pain away
Thank you for my nephew
I waited long to see
He was even more beautiful
Than I imagined him to be
I'm so glad I saw him
He looked so peaceful and sweet
It will stay with me forever
His little hands, and his little feet
You would have made an amazing mother
As everyone could see
With Michael as a dad
How fantastic you both would have been
The bond Edward shared with you
With all those kicks in your tum
I think I kind of know
After all, you were my second mum
Our Little Miss Sunshine
A ray of light so tall
Unbelievable brave
An Inspiration to us all
A wife and a sister
A daughter and a mother
How grateful and proud I am
To call myself your brother
Your light shone on so many

Everyone you met
The love you gave to us all
We will never forget
Two brothers have lost their sister
So this is why I say
For those of you with sisters
Love them more and more each day
The tears we cry, the pain we feel
Is because you have gone
We accept you're not coming back
But in our hearts you live on
Those words we shared on your last day
Have never been more true
So I end this tribute by saying
Dear Sally, I love you.

'MORE THAN WORDS CAN SAY'
by Graham Passey

I miss you dearest Sally
I miss you every day
I long to see your face once more
More than words can say
Thank you for the rainbows
Thank you for your smile
Thank you for the love we shared
For letting me walk you down the aisle
Thank you for the visits
That brightened up my day
For the cards, the calls, and messages
More than words can say
I know your smile will rescue me
Will melt away the pain
I will learn to see the benefits
Of both the sun and rain
I loved you like no other
So special in every way
Your smile could lift the darkest hour
More than words can say
I will never forget you
For a part of me has died
You are in every breath I take

And the tears I cried and cried
Thank you for my grandson
So brief his earthly stay
So bitter sweet the memories
More than words can say
When I think of all we shared
The joyful and the sad
You always make me proud to say
That I am Sally's dad
I know that you are in God's care
And of this I simply pray
May your light perpetual shine
More than words can say

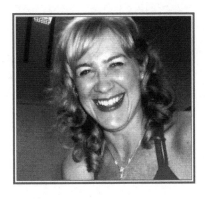

SALLY REMEMBERED

Sally was pure gold to the core.
Professor Elwyn Elias, co-founder of the Queen
Elizabeth transplant unit

To be called one of 'her boys' was a unique privilege.
Darius Mirza, consultant surgeon

*We are all richer for having known her, devastated that we
have lost her and determined that we shall never forget her.*
David Mayer, retired transplant surgeon

Sally was an angel sent from above who shone on all of us.
Pat Knight, hospital domestic

Sally was like a pot of gold at the end of a rainbow.
Nora Collins, hospital domestic

Friends are the family you choose for yourself.
Thank you so much for making me feel part of your
family, and thank you Sal for being you.
Sarah Cooper, family friend

Profits from the sale of this book will go to the Sally
Painting Memorial Fund, providing therapeutic
treatments to liver patients at the Queen Elizabeth
Hospital, Birmingham.